DEVELOPING RE PRACTICE

Making sense of social work in a world of change

Edited by Helen Martyn

With:

Michael Atkinson, Mary Cody, Jane Dutton, Veronique Faure, Rosemary Gordon, Patrick Kidner, Stephen Kitchman, Patrick Lonergan, Michael O'Dempsey, Sigurd Reimers and Kate Wilson

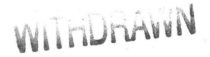

First published in Great Britain in June 2000 by

The Policy Press
University of Bristol
34 Tyndall's Park Road
Bristol BS8 1PY
UK

Tel +44 (0)117 954 6800
Fax +44 (0)117 973 7308
E-mail tpp@bristol.ac.uk
http://www.bristol.ac.uk/Publications/TPP

ISBN 1 86134 238 1

Helen Martyn was formerly Lecturer in Social Work, Goldsmiths College,
University of London.

The National Institute for Social Work receives support from the Department
of Health and aims to promote excellence in social work and social care. The
views expressed are those of the authors and not necessarily those of funding
bodies.

Front cover: Photograph supplied by kind permission of www.johnbirdsall.co.uk
Cover design by Qube Design Associates, Bristol
Printed in Great Britain by Hobbs the Printers Ltd, Southampton

Contents

Preface

Daphne Statham CBE

Developing reflective practice challenges a number of stereotypes about social work. Far from not having a knowledge base, the writers demonstrate that expert practitioners use a wide range of existing theories and methodologies. The writers, all students on Goldsmith College's Advanced Programme, also widened their theoretical base by accessing the expertise of other professionals. Like any experts they know when they do not have the skills to do the work unaided, and to take the initiative in supplementing what they know and can do.

As a result their expertise as social workers shines out. Far from being bound by organisational procedures, they were creative in tailoring their work to individual children and young people. The chapters show how social work can make a difference to the way young people face their pasts and live their futures.

The book provides a welcome resource for identifying what needs to be in place for social workers to become expert in what they do. This cannot be achieved without support from experienced colleagues and access to other professions. Good practice is essentially interprofessional and crosses organisational boundaries. This recognition has all too often been absent in recent years, when supervision has often concentrated on accountability for budgets and procedures.

Important though this is, it is not enough if we are to move from routine to skilled practice tailored to the specific support required by individual children and young people. The opportunity to reflect on practice is essential if social workers are to develop their expertise and provide services that are child and young people centred.

A second theme is that good practice cannot be sustained if social workers cannot face the pain of working with young people who have had severe and damaging experiences (DoH, 1988). The fact that without support most workers will not hear what young people are saying has been well established for many years. We ignore this knowledge to the peril of young people's futures. The Quality Protects initiative has made these futures the core business of organisations working with children and young people.

Social workers are important to young people: whether they are good or not matters to them. Both the young people and the social workers Jenny Morris interviewed agreed that neither was satisfied with what was happening. They mentioned lack of time, too many cases and not being listened to as things that blocked young people getting the support they expected from their social workers (Morris, 2000). Young people say that they want a relationship that demonstrates that what happens to them matters.

If workers are to achieve this, they must become committed to the young people they work with. There are consequences for social workers as well as for young people as a result of the fragmentation of services or organisational restructuring. Both will experience loss when the relationship ends or changes its basis. Successful outcomes are dependent on providing access to excellent, not indifferent or even mediocre, support for social workers.

Lifelong learning is an expectation for the population as a whole. The importance of continuing professional development being built into the careers of social workers is well demonstrated in each chapter of this book. Good intentions are insufficient. The skills secured in qualifying training can easily be degraded into what passes muster in the employing agency. Where standards are high, learning on the job will be a major source for improvement.

Equally, organisations that promote excellence will assume that this alone will not be enough. External expertise is a resource that needs to supplement, but not replace, learning from and alongside colleagues. Together these create a critical mass of expertise that can deliver the core business of the organisation: supporting children and young people in overcoming obstacles that have blocked their development, so that they can fulfil their potential and play their part in community life.

Finally, each chapter puts a nail in the coffin of the view that social work requires no more from those who practice it than learning how to be a 'streetwise granny'. Honourable though the role of grandmother is, and much as I love being one, the idea that being streetwise is sufficient is totally misconceived. The work is highly complex. The level of education and training required to do the work must rise not decrease, and post-qualifying and advanced learning has to become routine and not the exception.

This is something most social workers know is necessary and want. The students' work recorded in *Developing reflective practice*, and the outcomes for the children and young people they worked with, show that the investment of time and resources is well worthwhile.

Reflections, partnerships and teams: an acknowledgement

Helen Martyn

A reflection may be either a replica or a distortion of the original (as anyone who has visited Madame Tussaud's will know). A partnership requires a twosome, but rather than one side being an image or reflection of the other, the two may be quite different and the coming together the result of a common interest or shared commitment.

Developing reflective practice has resulted from a partnership, originally growing out of a developing relationship between Goldsmiths College and the National Institute for Social Work (NISW). Were it not for her reluctance, it would be attributed to a joint editorship, for without Margaret Hogan, Publications Manager at NISW, and the resources of NISW, most notably the technical assistance of Gary Parselle, this book would not have progressed from an idea to a reality. In acknowledging and thanking Margaret for her skilled and informed work and her enthusiastic commitment, I also want to say that like other productive partnerships, it has also been enjoyable.

Partnerships can extend into team work and this has also happened, most significantly with Patrick Kidner's involvement in planning the book as well as contributing the final chapter. Yet the bulk is written by six former members of the Goldsmiths Programme and the four commentators. My warmest thanks to each and all of them. And last, but by no means least, to my own partner Roger, whose staunch and tolerant support and willing involvement has helped to compensate for my technological, and other, inadequacies.

So it is that the work of a number of people from differing backgrounds with a range of knowledge and skills, occupying different positions and performing various roles, have come together to create *Developing reflective practice* out of a shared concern to promote effective social work practice with children and families.

Notes on contributors and commentators

Contributors

Michael Atkinson graduated with a BA (Hons) in sociology in 1981 and began working with children and families as a nursery officer for a London borough in 1983. From 1991 he managed a nursery in another borough, which was piloted as a children's centre and developed a broad range of services to families, including parenting groups. He currently manages a family resource centre offering support to looked-after children and families in need.

Mary Cody completed a social science degree at University College Dublin, then worked as part of a multi-disciplinary team in rural Ireland with a specific interest in child mental health. She then studied for the CQSW at Dundee University and now works in a specialist voluntary agency, where over the past 10 years she has been able to pursue her interests in working towards good outcomes for children and the permanent placement of children separated from their birth families.

Veronique Faure lived and studied in France where she gained a degree in sociology and a diploma in social work. Recruited to work for a London borough, she has 10 years' experience in childcare and child protection, both as a practitioner and a manager. She also has a certificate in counselling skills and the Goldsmiths diploma.

Stephen Kitchman has a BA (Hons) in sociology and gained his CQSW in 1989. He has since worked in the East End of London as a social worker, senior practitioner and team manager in statutory social services in both generic and specialist children and families teams. He is currently working as a child protection coordinator, studying the development of models of family decision making and increasing children's participation within the work of social services.

Patrick Lonergan qualified in 1979 with a CQSW, and in 1995 gained the Goldsmiths diploma. He worked as a generic social worker for a total of seven years. Since 1991 he has worked as a social worker in a children and families team in an inner London borough, and was previously a senior social worker in a permanency team for two years. He is currently a senior social worker in a children and families neighbourhood team in inner London.

Michael O'Dempsey emigrated to New Zealand after completing the Goldsmiths diploma. After a year working in a statutory child protection agency, he has worked for the Christchurch Methodist Mission Child and Family Services. This is largely a therapeutic, home-based social work service. Challenges in coming to practice in New Zealand have been new laws, new cultures (Maori, Pacific Island and Kiwi) and the developing culture of social work there.

Commentators

Jane Dutton is a Principal Lecturer in Social Work at Middlesex University. She is a UKCP registered systemic psychotherapist and supervisor, and a visiting tutor at the Tavistock Clinic where she contributes to a postgraduate family therapy training programme. Recent research and publications reflect a particular interest in working in diversity in social work and family therapy training.

Rosemary Gordon works for the NSPCC as a training manager for external services. Her background is in probation, where latterly she worked as a divorce court welfare officer before joining the NSPCC in 1986 as a child protection team manager.

Sigurd Reimers is a family therapist with Avon and Western Wiltshire Mental Health Care (NHS) Trust, and a training officer with Somerset Area Child Protection Committee. He previously worked as a social worker in an English psychiatric hospital, a Welsh social services area office, and British and Norwegian child and family guidance centres. He is the author, with Andy Treacher, of *Introducing user-friendly family therapy* (Routledge, 1995). For 10 years he wrote the social policy column for the family therapy news magazine *Context*.

Kate Wilson is a Senior Lecturer in Social Work at the University of York, where she teaches on the postgraduate MA programme in social work, and directs the University's post qualifying MA/Diploma programme in non-directive play therapy and the post qualifying childcare training programme for social workers. Her research interests are in fostering and adoption and in play therapy. Her *Case studies in non-directive play therapy* (with Virginia Ryan) has just been reprinted by Jessica Kingsley.

Final chapter

Patrick Kidner, after early experience in the probation service and social work teaching, joined Wandsworth Social Services Department in 1976 as a team manager. He then held several more senior posts, most recently that of district manager (children and families) until 1997. He now works on a freelance basis with local authorities and voluntary organisations, mainly on issues relating to child protection and looked after children.

Editor

Helen Martyn was Lecturer in Social Work at Goldsmiths College, University of London, 1975-97, where for the last 15 years she had lead responsibility for the Advanced Social Work Programme. She is currently involved in the management of a church-based social work agency and is chair of an adoption panel in an inner London authority.

Introduction

Helen Martyn

This is a book about social work practice with children and families. As such it is one of many, and as many do, it focuses on the elusive but necessary search for effective practice. But what distinguishes this volume from others is that it is based on assessed work submitted on a post-qualifying programme which aimed to develop the practice skills of experienced social workers. It is thus illustrative of the actual dilemmas, struggles and rewards of practice in the late 1990s. The work is mostly drawn from the statutory sector.

The format adopted mirrors the process of the programme, where the rigours and realities of practice entered vividly into the classroom, not solely as illustration or even anecdote, but as the true fabric of learning. When the practice accounts were read and the research analysed it was the users, and particularly the young users, of services who were the pivot of attention. And it is the users who are central to this book. The course members who worked with them present here their attempts to intervene helpfully. This work in turn is analysed by four independent commentators.

I will outline the programme, state how this book came about in the form it has, comment on its intended usefulness and then go on to discuss some themes of contemporary relevance.

The Programme

The Postgraduate Diploma in Advanced Social Work (Children and Families) was set up in 1983 at Goldsmiths College, University of London, where a well-regarded one-year postgraduate CQSW course was already established. The Programme came about from a shared concern in the multi-disciplinary education committee of British Agencies for Adoption and Fostering (BAAF) about current standards of social work practice. The roots of this Programme were therefore in practice; they were interdisciplinary (law, medicine, child psychiatry, as well as social work); and they were about raising standards. These themes remained constant throughout the 14 years of the Programme's existence. The people

xi

involved remained constant also, most notably two members of that education committee, Margaret Adcock and Richard White, whose teaching was central to the curriculum.

The Programme took place over an academic year, with 55 teaching days in college and a roughly equivalent time for completion of the practice component of the course. This took place in the course member's employing agency and centred on specified areas of practice: direct work with children and work with a family were two such areas. It is these which provide the material for this book.

Each course member had a designated practice coordinator (usually a senior member of the agency staff) whose responsibility it was to ensure that the Programme's practice requirement could be met, to provide some or all of the practice supervision, and then coordinate the final report. The provision existed for some supervision to be subcontracted to specialist staff. The current trend to place increasing responsibility for assessment of practice on employing agencies was thus foreshadowed.

This system also resulted in some variations in practice, over which the College had little control in spite of clearly stated criteria. Some course members were clearly better served than others: the implications of this are commented on in the work which follows. The individual course member's tutor was responsible for facilitating these arrangements and for integrating the course member's learning from college and agency. Three-way agency-based meetings were held throughout the programme, a necessary but expensive procedure. Course members remained in employment throughout, so the contracted practice agreement at the outset of the Programme was essential.

Satellite programmes

The course was favourably received by most employing agencies, several of whom seconded staff on a regular basis. One such authority, Kent County Council, decided to set up its own satellite programme in 1987 and three years later a third programme followed at NCH Action for Children; the latter also admitted social workers from other agencies. A fuller account of these programmes and an evaluation of their outcome can be found in Rushton and Martyn (1993). The Kent Programme continued until 1994 when it moved to Christ's College, Canterbury. The NCH Action for Children Programme ran for the four years as planned. The Goldsmiths Programme, much dented by changes in the structure and funding of post-qualifying education (CCETSW, 1992), as well as by Higher Education policies and funding constraints in general, closed in 1997.

Other publications

Raising standards should also involve raising awareness. Much has been published by individual course members themselves over the years, but this book is the third publication based on course-related practice. Each is different in structure and focus, although all three share a concern to analyse and promote effective social work practice. *Direct work with children* (Aldgate and Simmonds, 1988) was based on work submitted in the early years of the course and sought to enable and enthuse social workers to develop interest and skill in the then less known area of direct work with children. *Working with children in need* (Sainsbury, 1994) was a more substantial volume which identified and discussed a range of current themes, such as the experience of sexual abuse, social work across racial, cultural and language differences, and presented these as studies in complexity and challenge.

Developing reflective practice: making sense of social work in a world of change

The intention of this book is to present vivid examples of social work practice with children and families which provide, not necessarily exemplars of skilled intervention but, more usefully, real life illustrations of the challenges now facing practitioners. The Programme at Goldsmiths was constantly seeking ways to develop more effective practice. To achieve the same purpose here, we invited both educators and practitioners to provide analytic commentaries on the presented work, indicating what went well, what not so well, and where improvements might have been made. Thus social work practice in all its pain and complexity, as well as its potential for growth, change and empowerment, forms the core of this work.

Developing reflective practice is mostly based on work submitted in the final year of the course when confidence had grown to the point where it was possible to expose work to rigorous analysis and criticism from outside commentators. The choice of material was not easily made. We have tried to select work which demonstrates a range of practice situations and methods of intervention. As will be apparent, we did not set out to present the work of six star performers, although we believe that much of this work is both accomplished and vividly presented. This said, it is no small risk for any professional person to expose the fine detail of their work to external analysis and then to a wide readership. If other workers can be helped to develop their practice and if users thereby receive a more effective service as a result of this book, then it is the six social workers from the Goldsmiths Programme (five of whom are currently practising in and around London) who must be thanked most of all.

The course organisers were continually indebted to a number of eminent people in many ways, but most particularly in the formal teaching programme. It might have seemed natural to turn to some of them for analytic commentaries. We did not do this. Most established programmes of study develop their own culture (and the Goldsmiths course seemed to develop a particularly powerful one), so it was therefore important to seek other equally eminent people 'outside the family' to do this work for us. None of the commentators have any formal link with the course, although it is fair to say that they had different levels of awareness of it through their own networks. They were chosen as independent and knowledgeable people whose reputations were established through their writing and other professional activities. None of them knew each other beyond this.

Each commentator wrote their analysis independently, and, although scripts were later exchanged, no significant amendments were made or requested. We were therefore pleased, but not surprised, to see some quite different points made. While there is little frank disagreement, there are clear differences of emphasis as well as areas of overlap. The commentators were all equally concerned with effectiveness and do not always reach consensus as to what constitutes it.

Practice cannot and does not take place in a vacuum, but in increasingly tightly managed agency settings. It was thus essential to have a concluding chapter written from a management perspective. In his days as an area director of an inner London social services department, Patrick Kidner enabled a number of staff to study on the Programme. By his active encouragement of staff to develop their practice skills, it was clear that Patrick was not one of those managers who was prepared to accept that this necessarily means 'You are not a social worker now' (Kearney and Rosen, 1999). So it was to him that we turned for the manager's perspective. An added bonus was Patrick's willingness to join some of our planning and editorial discussions.

The structure of the book

Developing reflective practice is divided into two main sections: the first focuses on direct work with children, and the second on work with families. The analytic commentaries follow the case material. Each section has a brief introduction and a list of learning points at the end. The concluding chapter is written from a management perspective.

Readership

The book provides guidance for both students (on how to realise practice in a coursework context) and teachers (on how to assess coursework and enhance student practice). It will also be of relevance for practitioners (on how to approach specific pieces of work) and managers and supervisors (on how to promote best practice). While the practice illustrations as 'narrative' may arouse the interest of those considering entering professional social work training, the analytic discourse, based as it is on a substantial theoretical base, provides a vital initiation into the theoretical underpinnings of social work practice. Finally it is hoped that those studying for post-qualifying and advanced awards in social work, especially when working to complete modules in relative isolation, will find *Developing reflective practice* and its extensive references an invaluable resource.

This book aims, in essence, to establish standards for both education and practice rooted in the reality of the workplace. There is not, so far as we are aware, any publication which takes this approach or uses course material in its original form, thus preserving and capitalising on actual lived experience as a source of reflection.

Reflective and effective practice

The themes of reflective practice and effective practice resonate and recur throughout this book: ideally they are two sides of the same coin. If there was one process which the course teaching sought to challenge, it was the stimulus/reaction/action response rather than stimulus/reflection/action. Effectiveness commonly resides in the difference between reaction and reflection, as long as it is informed reflection. The case material which follows attempts to demonstrate this. Yet reflection is not just an individual process: it also needs support and encouragement, as Patrick Kidner addresses in the final chapter. At best, reflective practice needs a culture, an environment, in which to take root and flourish.

Thirty years ago Ronald Laing gave a paper to the Association of Family Caseworkers in what Dame Eileen Younghusband described as "the beguiling and imaginative English in which Dr Laing so gently leads us out of our depth".

In stressing the need for both psychiatrists and social workers to be practical, Laing went on to say:

> We have hectic jobs; our theorising is often done in the midst of our activity, or in our spare time when we are not too exhausted. We often discover what we do after we have done it. An advantage of this is a certain empirical pragmatic approach. Disadvantages are that without time for critical reflection we may become dogmatic in theory and keep repeating ourselves in practice. We may even keep repeating a story about what we repetitiously do which does not even match what we do; especially if we do not have sufficient time to scrutinise what we are actually doing. (Laing, 1969, p 4)

In the work which follows there is abundant evidence of earlier repetitious reaction (see, for example, Carol's history). It is all too easy for social workers to become institutionalised into a certain routinised response and indeed, the culture of some practice agencies seems to reinforce this in a powerful and compelling way. This process can be as stultifying for workers caught up in it as it is limiting and disrespectful to users on the receiving end of the service.

One of the common motivations for experienced social workers applying to the Goldsmiths (and doubtless other) programmes was that they felt 'bogged down', 'stuck', at risk of burn-out. Most committed practitioners in the helping professions are aware, even if not always very consciously so, when their work lacks creativity, sensitivity, thoughtfulness and energy. In these situations it is well nigh impossible to hear the messages being conveyed, let alone respond adequately to them. So it is that the service which individual users receive is heavily dependent on the staff delivering it, which in turn depends on the policies, practices and general state of play in the employing agency. A clearly unacceptable state of affairs.

If it seems depressing to recognise that words spoken over 30 years ago still resonate powerfully today, it is equally important to interject a note of optimism and to recognise positive trends and developments since then. There has been an explosion in the relevant knowledge base; *Developing reflective practice* is intended to assist access to it. Research activity has gathered pace and some good examples focus on the study of effectiveness: see, for example, Sainsbury et al, 1982, Rees and Wallace, 1982, Sheldon, 1986, Cheetham et al, 1992, McDonald et al, 1992, Harding and Beresford, 1996. There is a greatly increased emphasis on accountability, more rigorous quality assurance and inspection procedures: the imminent creation of the General Social Care Council (Brand, 1999), to establish uniform standards, and the proposed Social Care Institute for Excellence now under discussion, to give guidance on good practice, should eventually provide social work with a firm foundation for practice and its management.

At the launch of the Greater London Post Qualifying Consortium in the early 1990s a triumphant note was sounded: 'every practice agency a learning environment'. An eminently laudable goal, but how lamentably far from reality. 'Quality Protects', a recent government initiative tells us (DoH, 1998b). Maybe. But social work is rarely a stand-alone activity, and has to find its position in a complex web of structures, policies, philosophies and relationships, all of which have to be taken into account as well as the intangible goal of 'quality'.

Social work needs public recognition and respect. In the research on effectiveness cited above, frequent reference is made to the tendency for negative evaluations to be publicly disseminated rather than positive outcomes. Cheetham et al (1992) write:

> Much of the interest and worth of social work lies in its contribution to alleviating the enduring problems of poverty, ill-health, disability, struggling and disintegrating relationships. But since the responses to such troubles are often both contentious and ill-resourced, social work by its association with them can reap the whirlwind. (Cheetham et al, 1992, p 145)

Patrick Kidner sensibly questions the wisdom of the profession so openly displaying its limitations. The risk is acknowledged and only seems acceptable in the quest for articulating, and hopefully attaining, higher, and uniformly higher, standards of practice. A (moderately) sympathetic journalist once wrote that doctors bury their mistakes, but social workers generally have to live with theirs.

Social work practice and management: a symbiotic relationship?

> The primacy of practice, its development and the maintenance of good practice standards should be robustly promoted by the wider organisation. (Cheetham et al, 1992, p 20)

NISW's Management of Practice Expertise Project (Rosen, 2000) is focused on just this task. In the preface to the Project report, Denise Platt, Chief Inspector of the Social Services Inspectorate at the Department of Health, writes "I believe strongly that this neglected area must have the attention it deserves, because service quality depends on it." Yet, as Patrick Kidner discusses in the final chapter of this book, the relationship between social work practice and its management is, at best, an uneasy one:

> There is a real danger that the creative role of practitioners will be stifled by increasingly bureaucratic and prescriptive forms of management if more attention is not urgently given to the support and development of first-line managers and practice supervisors.

Rosen (2000) explores the tendency to split social work management and practice into separate discrete activities, more readily than to identify common ground. They write:

> The conventional wisdom is that managers are recruited as 'expert practitioners' and then need to 'leave practice' or 'give up being a practitioner' and learn to be 'managers'. Although we recognise that managers need to develop their capacity to manage, this conventional 'wisdom' is seriously flawed.... (p 16)

> It is a myth that good practice and good management inhabit different worlds – both involve working with people to achieve tasks, to solve complex problems, or to manage those that are insoluble, and to achieve change in social situations and relationships. (p 16)

Such a split between social work management and practice and the consequent constraint in transferring skills can only be to the detriment of both groups of workers and therefore, most significantly, to the service individual service users receive. This split also throws light on the reluctance many employing agencies expressed about releasing senior staff to study on the Goldsmiths Programme: such senior people should surely be looking to management courses. At least some other professions enable their most highly trained and experienced staff to undertake the most complex work. This should be a central concern in social work. Until the relationship between social work practice and its management is satisfactorily resolved, it seems unlikely that the ambivalence which Patrick Kidner describes at the end of his chapter will diminish.

It is all too easy for practitioners to criticise those managers who impose tasks on them and fail to provide the conditions in which creative and effective practice can take place. Pressures are exerted on first-line managers from above; hence the value of the "vertical slice work" developed in the NISW Project to "tackle some key issues and debrief about the development of practice activities" (Kearney, 1999, p 19). What seems to be necessary is shared identification with a common and clearly defined task, whereby front-line staff, including administrative staff, and their middle and senior managers are together committed to delivering a high quality service. They also need to be clear about the boundaries of role necessary to achieve this aim.

Singing from the same hymn sheet can sound melodious whether the singing is in unison or in harmony. To push this analogy further, an agency needs to be in unison in respect of its aims, but the means of achieving them involve harmony, with different groups 'singing' different parts which together create a pleasing sound. There has to be mutual trust, between all participants, that colleagues have the skill and confidence to hold their own line if the perils of discordant collapse are to be avoided.

To return to social work:

> Organisations taking on the corporate parenting of children and the care of vulnerable people need to be beacons of the integrity that fosters high levels of trust. Where managers and workers distrust each other, avoiding blame takes the place of taking responsibility. (Rosen, 2000, p 5)

In the light of the pressure on local authority social services departments in particular to provide a range of services as economically as possible, it may seem tempting for managers to require front-line staff to close down work in the hope that it will go away, or go somewhere else, rather than open it up and either work towards a resolution of the problem or identify, with the user, a more manageable way of living with it: in Sigurd Reimer's analysis, to move away from the 'explorer' role.

Those social workers entering the Goldsmiths Programme over the years would echo Kearney's (1999) account of the views of the participants in the NISW Project, that "the development of practice expertise has become a 'closet activity'. For example, advanced practice training was often undertaken at the worker's expense with little support and even overt hostility from managers" (see also Rushton and Martyn, 1993, p 7). The complementary activities of social work practice and its management need to come out of the closet into the open – where they may attract public recognition.

And – into a world of change

The subtitle of *Developing reflective practice* implies that it is indeed possible for social work to make sense while the world is changing – although there can be few in the field who have not had reason to doubt this from time to time! Looking ahead into the new millennium, much remains unclear. Yet if one thing is certain it is that change is a continual process. It is not going to stop happening, however fervently we may sometimes wish it. The profession would therefore be well advised to divert energy invested in trying to resist change into developing the knowledge and skill to live with it, and be stimulated by it.

Not everything has to change all the time. Perhaps people and the way they relate to each other do not change that much; but social situations change and evolve, as do the social and political influences that determine them. Change needs to be planned and managed if social work is to make sense (Smale, 1999). Beyond that, the extent to which the processes can be understood and accepted, the more possible it should become to identify and work with them. This may be easy to say, but it is a complex and often anxiety laden experience to live through.

In her seminal work in relation to the organisation of nursing services, Menzies wrote:

> Change is inevitably, to some extent, an excursion into the unknown. It implies a commitment to future events that are not entirely predictable and to their consequences, and inevitably provokes doubt and anxiety. Any significant change within a social system implies changes in existing social relationships and in social structure. It follows that any significant social change implies a change in the operation of the social system as a defence system. While this change is proceeding, ie while social defences are being re-structured, anxiety is likely to be more open and intense. (Menzies, 1970, p 22)

Thirty years later Kearney lists surviving re-re-organisation as one of the key elements in managing change and innovation (Kearney, 1999). There is undeniably a need for periodic review of the structures and methods of delivery of social work services. However, it is worth reflecting where the thrust for successive rounds of re-organisation comes from and to question, in Menzies' (1970) analysis, whether it might relate to the anxiety inevitably generated by the task; that is, by social work's necessary identification with troubled and troubling people and situations. This anxiety is experienced both institutionally (in the way organisations function) and by the individuals and groups that form the organisation. If social work is to make more sense in a changing world, the understanding of, training for, and management of, change is of fundamental importance.

Change involves loss (Marris, 1974); social workers should have finely honed skills to help users survive a whole range of loss experiences. A similar level of understanding and skill needs to be applied to·the organisations in which social workers are employed. In this way the more open and intense anxiety which Menzies refers to could be recognised and addressed.

Reference has already been made in this introduction to the need for clear standards of good practice and Laing's (1969) emphasis on the need for social workers (and psychiatrists) to be practical. Some of the most public, and I believe justifiable, criticisms of social work relate to tolerance of standards of living that most would find unacceptable, if not frankly abhorrent. An explanation, but by no means an excuse, for this might well lie in the familiarity many social workers have with modes and styles of living which are at best unsatisfactory and at worst seriously neglectful and abusive. As Jane Dutton writes, "In the social work context, the extraordinary may become ordinary".

If social work is to be seen to make sense then it needs to locate the authority to make well informed and clearly evidenced professional judgements which resonate with society's values, as expressed by the law and policy and practice guidelines. In this way the extraordinary can be recognised for what it is and action taken, rather than being tolerated as ordinary and left unchallenged.

One of the most powerful and necessary developments in recent decades has been the recognition and development of anti-discriminatory and anti-oppressive practice (regrettably, still rather patchily applied). Vital as this is, it could be that a misconception of anti-discriminatory practice has inhibited both some social workers and some agencies from setting appropriate standards in order to protect vulnerable members of society. At worst, this can lead to dangerous practice which is itself discriminatory (consider, for example, the deaths of a number of black children, such as Jasmine Beckford [Blom-Cooper et al, 1985] and Kimberley Carlile [Blom-Cooper et al, 1987]). If social work is to make sense, it needs continually to seek to articulate, in an informed and sensitive way, what is and what is not acceptable. This is not just a task for social work. It needs to be the subject of dialogue and wider debate.

It is entirely proper for social work, and any other professional activity, to be accountable to society. In order to do this social work needs to state its aims clearly and unambiguously, explain some of its processes, and set its standards. In this way it has a chance of making sense not only to its users, but also to its workers and managers and through them to society at large. Our hope and intention is that *Developing reflective practice* can make a useful contribution to this process.

Part 1:
Direct work with children and young people

Introduction

Helen Martyn

> It is the responsibility of adults to develop the possibilities for children
> and so secure a better future for us all. (Cattenach, 1992, p 10)

On first reading this does not seem to be a particularly controversial statement, for it is self-evident that the dependency of all immature beings requires responsible care and nurture from those in situations of power and relative maturity. If only chronological age and emotional development were more closely aligned, then adults would be in a better position to exercise responsibility, gain satisfaction and pleasure from doing so, and thus open up the 'better future' for all.

This quotation is notable for its implicit message that adequate responses to the needs of the young are in the interests of adults as well as children. In the last analysis it could be argued that the needs of all generations lie along the same axis, yet examples abound where the needs of children and adults have become divergent rather than convergent. This creates a space full of pain and confusion where social workers and others have to operate.

It was part of the fundamental philosophy of the Goldsmiths course that while the needs of adults should always be attended to, the child is central. The Children Act (1989) has enshrined this principle (Section 1.1), although some of the interpretations of the legislation (for example DoH, 1993, paras 2.19 to 2.21, DoH, 1994, paras 2.25, 2.26) may have obscured this focus, a point further discussed later in this section.

Given the range and depth of social work responsibility for children and young people in need or at risk, it is disturbing that much qualifying training has given somewhat scant regard to developing knowledge and skill in direct work with them. A growing body of literature in the last decade (for example, Aldgate and Simmonds, 1988; Batty, 1989; Cattenach, 1992, 1994; Sainsbury, 1994; West, 1996) and curriculum developments in the Diploma in Social Work (Dip SW) (CCETSW, 1995) are going some way to address this omission. Even so, it is largely in post-qualifying education and training that this provision is made, both through a range of shorter inhouse courses, or on longer external programmes such as that at the University of York referred to later by Kate Wilson.

Direct work teaching: relevance and limitation

So it was that many experienced practitioners came to the Goldsmiths course with little knowledge or skill in direct work and even an anxiety (if not a fear) of it (see Stephen Kitchman's comments in his account of work with Carol). The course was fortunate to secure the services of a number of external trainers to teach a short, specific three-day sequence, which was then supplemented by work in other parts of the teaching programme, in seminar, tutorial and supervisory work.

Such limited training could only give an introduction to this huge and complex subject. It is arguable that, without more time or resources, the attempt to teach and assess direct work should not have been attempted at all. Yet over and against this, it would be a serious dereliction of responsibility if any programme with 'advanced social work with children and families' in its title did not seek to develop standards of work with children. The child is properly at the centre of all intervention, even if it is not always possible or appropriate to work directly with them.

It may be a searingly obvious point to make (yet successive child abuse enquiry reports bear testament to its neglect: DoH, 1991a), but adults charged with responsibility for children all too readily lose sight of the child, as they become consumed by their own internal and external dynamics: this can be true of parents, carers or professionals. It is often easier for adults to make a more ready identification with other adults, rather than with children. In her introduction (see p 87) Rosemary Gordon states that one of her current interests is the exploration of conceptions of childhood and how these are played out in the systems and structures we employ with them.

It can be emotionally costly and anxiety provoking to observe children: it frequently locates the needy defenceless child in the adult observer. Again, a recent body of literature (for example, Trowell and Miles, 1991; Wilson, 1992; Briggs, 1992; Le Riche and Tanner, 1998) raises awareness and develops our understanding. Limited child observation was a requirement of the Goldsmiths course, as it now also is on some qualifying programmes (for example, at Goldsmiths College and the University of York).

So what could we hope to achieve with this brief teaching sequence? Certainly an encouragement to enter the emotional life of the child:

both commentators note evidence of this in the work that follows. The course aimed to provide an introduction to methods of observation, assessment and intervention. The formal assessment requirements included evidence of practice in five elements of work: direct work with a child aged under 12, and work with a family. The five pieces of work which follow were two of these. They are of varying length as they relate to different assessment requirements.

Theoretical basis of the work

The main theoretical bases informing this work are attachment theory (Bowlby, 1971, 1979; Fahlberg, 1981a; Main, 1991; Bretherton, 1991; Howe, 1995), post-traumatic stress theory (Van der Kelk et al, 1987; Briere, 1992), and child development theory (Winnicot, 1964; Pringle, 1975; Stewart et al, 1985; Tizard, 1987), all informed by and filtered through sharp awareness of issues of race and culture, gender and other difference, and a clear commitment to empowerment. The work which follows is fully referenced: the centrality of attachment theory is clear.

Context of the work

Much of the literature on direct work rightly stresses the importance of appropriate conditions in which the work can be effective. Several of the contributors were acutely aware that conditions in their agencies were far from ideal, and only took the risk of embarking on the work after thorough consultation with senior management, external consultants and colleagues (see, for example, Veronique Faure's work with Sarah). Even then, as Kate Wilson discusses in her commentary, there may be different views about the wisdom of starting this work. Here it should be noted that it was not always appropriate for course purposes to document fully other areas of the agency's work.

The roles of the link worker, where children were in substitute family care, and of the family's social worker are critical. As in Michael O'Dempsey's work with Amos and Christopher, agency policy and practice sometimes dictates that the same worker had to combine different roles. Nowhere is this combination of roles more problematic than where the child's 'therapeutic' worker is also the key worker, with responsibility to monitor and address child protection concerns. This was also an issue in Veronique Faure's work with Sarah.

In an ideal world it would clearly be preferable to defer undertaking direct therapeutically orientated work until such time as the child is in a stable situation, and carers and others in the child's environment are prepared for and supportive of the work. Yet a child's life goes on, often in highly unpredictable circumstances. It is therefore preferable for a concerned adult to stand alongside the child, to be tuned into their needs and responses, to offer an experience of adult attention and respect. Such respect must be characterised by sensitive attention to pacing and boundaries. This is a feature of all the work which follows, most particularly in Mary Cody's work with Eve and Michael O'Dempsey's with Amos and Christopher.

The legal framework

Legal intervention is increasingly a feature of local authority work with children. The Children Act (1989) requires that the "ascertainable wishes and feelings of the child concerned (considered in the light of his age and understanding)" (Section 1(3)(a)) are issues for the court to take into account in its decision making. As Rosemary Gordon reminds us, asking the child, for example, which parent they would prefer to live with is entirely inadequate, unfair and over–simplistic. Finely honed skills are required if the court is to be well informed.

This was one of the aims of Michael O'Dempsey's work, which also graphically illustrates the unpredictable and unanticipated course of events (separation of the foster carers, guardian *ad litem's* illness and withdrawal), which cruelly reflected the bitter volatility of the warring relationship of the birth parents. This can readily add to the children's underlying fear of and anxiety about their own fantasised destructive power.

All the children and young people discussed in Part 1 had some involvement with the legal process, but questions arise about the timeliness of legal intervention. Was Sarah's mother, with her own history of negligent parenting, given too many chances to demonstrate her adequacy as a parent? From the account here this commentator, at least, would suggest that had Sarah been removed earlier and placed for adoption like her older siblings, she would now be a happier and less damaged child. Her mother, particularly if given appropriate help, might also have had a better chance of a more satisfying life, if spared the experience of further abusing and rejecting her daughter. Here is an illustration of the Cattenach (1992) quote which opens this section.

Assessment skills of the highest order are needed if drift and its attendant damage are to be prevented. As Mary Cody states, reviewing Eve's earlier history, "seven years to say, yes, something terrible is happening to this child and it must stop". Yet the account of Carol's succession of placement moves and constant crises poses the question, was this 'care' from the state much less abusive than life in her birth family, or just different but equally so?

In the early 1990s when the Children Act was new, much emphasis was placed on working with the birth family and the 'no order' principle. The 1992 *Children Act report* (DoH, 1993) quotes a Social Services Inspectorate study and Departmental discussion which revealed a belief that local authorities had to demonstrate that working in partnership had broken down, or been exhausted, before a statutory order could be made. It goes on to state unequivocally that "this was not the intention of the legislation" (DoH, 1993, para 2.21, p 19). Partnership is thus presented more as a philosophy underpinning intervention, rather than a particular sequence of action (or more commonly inaction) in which children's needs and interests could be obscured, if not neglected.

We do not know James' mother's feelings at the time the care order was made, but it should be noted that eight years later, as James approached independent living, Patrick Lonergan was able to end his work as James' social worker throughout this time by having a meal with James and his mother. Partnership and legal action to protect children's interests are not, and should not be, mutually exclusive activities.

The need for assessment, containment and planning

When feelings run deep in a context of highly charged anxiety and risk, there is an increased danger of hasty reaction rather than careful reflection and analysis, both by the worker and, more broadly, in the helping network. Kate Wilson provides a timely reminder that assessment is a critical and necessary stage if intervention is to be effective. Yet assessment is an ongoing process which needs to be continually reviewed and revised as work progresses; a sound assessment can also involve therapeutic gains, as demonstrated in, for example, Michael O'Dempsey's work with Amos and Christopher.

So it is that the need for intellectual rigour, organisational efficiency and careful planning is heightened by the emotional intensity of the work. Frameworks, as well as the people and structures that support them, can help contain anxiety and chaos. Older children, such as Carol, Eve and James, can be empowered by helping to negotiate the frameworks. Such simple procedures as agreeing dates and times (and keeping them), sending copy letters where appropriate, help disempowered young people to feel more grown up and responsible – and can also encourage them to behave in the same way.

Much of the course teaching focused on the development of practice skills in direct communication with children; much of the class work was experiential and supported and informed by reading. Yet however brilliant and inspired the therapeutic insights, the work is unlikely to be useful unless it is carefully planned. Many of the children and young people using social work services have lives characterised by loss, lack, neglect, inconsistency, and, often, a pattern of failed and rejecting relationships. Social workers therefore need to work doubly hard to ensure that they do not replicate similar experiences with the young users of their services, by unknowingly triggering these recollections.

Both commentators refer to Stephen Kitchman's work with Carol as a positive example of effective planning, efficiently and painstakingly executed. The easy (and utterly unsatisfactory) alternative would have been to continue the pattern of reactive crisis-driven work, and thereby add another section to the volume of illegible records – and then preside over further failed placements beyond the ten Carol had already been in and out of during the preceding 10 months.

It should be noted that in order to try to break the previous pattern of poor practice it was necessary to secure management agreement. Time well invested in the short term is infinitely more satisfying for the worker, as well as effective for the users, than time absorbed in crisis work over months and years. As Kate Wilson comments, "the time and resources required must, at the time, have seemed considerable, but are negligible in comparison with what would have been required had the placement broken down, as must at one time have seemed likely".

Personal and professional boundaries

Reference was made earlier in this section to the emotional demands on the worker, and the reflections between the angry needy children being worked with and the inner life of the worker. Patrick Lonergan shares his own personal pain and professional distress in describing how his personal situation got in the way of his planned work with James and gave rise to "unexpectedly enormous emotional feelings". One of the commentators refers to this as "a flawed piece of work"; yet even flawed work, if this is what this was, can be retrieved, and have value for the user as well as rich learning for the worker. Readers will reach their own judgement about this.

In the last analysis, becoming a professional worker does not obliterate human frailty. It remains a vital professional responsibility to address boundary issues in order to be available to users, but there are situations where users may gain something from our frailties as well as our strengths. The role of supervision is crucial in order for an appropriate boundary to be discerned, reviewed and maintained.

Effectiveness: a subjective or objective reality?

As stated in the introduction, the two commentators were sent the five scripts and asked to write critical appraisals of the work. It is interesting to note where there was convergence, and where divergence, of views, most particularly in relation to effectiveness. There are, for example, markedly different analyses of Mary Cody's work with Eve. Is this the product of quite separate theoretical positions which in turn inform choice of methods of intervention? Or could it be that the boundary between social work and more frankly therapeutic approaches is differently interpreted?

There may be other explanations, and these could relate to agency function and/or supervisory input. Assessment of effectiveness undoubtedly has much to do with where the assessor is coming from in terms of values, theoretical orientation and experience. This was an issue sometimes keenly experienced on the practice panel of the Goldsmiths course, one more reflection of how complex it is to define effective social work practice.

User perspectives on effectiveness, often expressed in terms of satisfaction, should no more be ignored than uncritically accepted as a definitive judgement. There is now a growing literature on the subject, although understandably this is more developed in work with adult users of social work services (for example, Balloch, 1998). However, it should not be forgotten that seven-year-old Christopher, not liking himself or his name, wanted to be called Michael, like his social worker. Thirteen-year-old Carol surprised Stephen Kitchman by lighting a candle for him. How often do social workers permit themselves to acknowledge their significance to (particularly) young users? Equally importantly, if agencies allowed themselves to recognise the value of some of their front-line staff to the users of their service, would they be more constrained in reorganising at such perilously regular intervals? (See Kearney, 1999.)

The five accounts of practice follow with analytic commentaries. A list of learning points concludes the section.

Case studies

James:
Moving on to independent living

Patrick Lonergan

Context and purpose of the intervention

James is a 17-year-old young man of white British/Sicilian origin, currently in a long-term foster placement in North London with a single white female carer, Mrs Appleby, who is in her mid–fifties and of white British origin. James is subject to a Section 31 care order under the Children Act (1989). He has been with his current carer for four years. It is expected that James will leave his current placement in six to 12 months and move on to semi or independent living. In my borough there is an independent living team (ILP) who undertake this work, so the case was due to be transferred.

I have been James' social worker for nearly eight years, so in transferring the case I wanted to do a piece of work lasting approximately three months around 'endings'. I discussed the work with James and we agreed that we would spend the sessions looking at his files, as I thought it was important for James to be able to make sense of early life events in relation to his current perception of himself and others.

In doing this it was envisaged that there would be some overlap with the formal transfer of the case which was due to take place shortly. James had already met his new social worker from the ILP and he had also had some contact with another member of the team, who helps young people with careers and employment, so we had already started preparing in a task centred way for the transfer (see Figure 1).

Assessment

I was aware from discussion with James that in commencing this work, he was ambivalent about having a new social worker, because in his understanding he was still subject to a care order for another 12 months. In my authority, in common with most local authorities, there is an expectation that young people being 'looked after' have to move on to semi or independent living between the ages of 16 and 18 years. Given that I had been his social worker for such a long period, I also knew that I would be sorry and sad to transfer the case. For me, working with James and his mother had become very satisfying and I was anxious to have a good handover to the ILP.

Unlike many adolescents I have known, James' experience of the care system was pretty positive. Given that he had spent nearly half his life being 'looked after', I felt a tremendous responsibility therefore, almost like a father figure, handing over the work to another section of the department. My experience of living and working in London and of research (Stein and Carey, 1986) is that a disproportionate number of single homeless young people have been 'looked after'. I remember thinking I did not want this to happen to James.

I thought that there would be two key aspects to the work: (i) issues of separation and loss, and (ii) transitions, because he was not only changing social worker, but moving towards independence, and from leaving college to seeking full-time employment.

Figure 1: Genogram

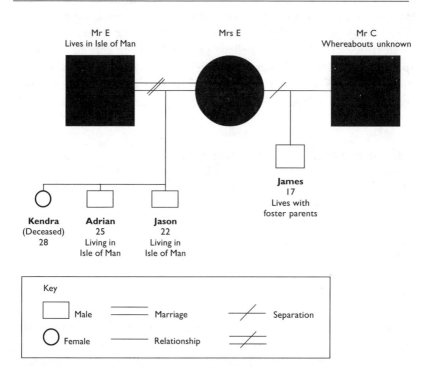

At the beginning of this piece of work, I negotiated extra time with my manager as I was proposing to see James fortnightly to do the sessions. I had agreed with James that he would come to the office. I also spoke to his foster carer, Mrs Appleby, and the ILP social worker about the work. I tried to see James' mother before the sessions commenced but was unable to, as she failed the appointment.

Theory

The theory I used in this case was chiefly drawn from psychoanalytic thinking and frameworks.

Attachment

Bowlby's work on attachment (1980), while being seen as important in understanding child–parent relationships, is criticised for its over-emphasis on maternal deprivation and the resulting damaging long-term consequences for children. Rutter (1972) states that studies of late adopted children show marked social and behavioural improvements. Rutter suggests we have to examine other environmental and social factors in order to reach a better understanding of how some children like James can overcome poor early parenting experiences.

In James' case, I strongly believe that he has been able to overcome poor early childhood experiences. This is not to say that James is a well adjusted adolescent, but I would suggest that he has physically and emotionally matured in recent years, particularly in exhibiting self-control.

Identity and adolescent development

Triseliotis (1983) identifies three important areas which contribute to identity building in adolescence: (i) having a childhood experience of feeling wanted and loved; (ii) knowledge of one's personal history; and (iii) the experience of being perceived by others as a worthwhile person. I hoped my direct work would help James with the latter two areas.

Separation and loss

I found Claudia Jewett's (1984) writing on 'endings' useful in that she describes how 'separation from the helper' should be gradual and planned. This process I hoped would allow James to express his feelings, and I wanted to give James a say in the ending of our relationship; thus we agreed to look at his past files, particularly the ones that covered pre-adolescence. I hoped in approaching it in this way we would both be involved in a period of healthy mourning so that James could move on and establish a relationship with his new worker in the ILP.

Process of the work

As I have said, I envisaged that this work with James would take approximately three months. In fact it took six. I propose, therefore, to focus only on selected sessions in this section. Soon after commencing the work, I was to suffer my own significant loss when my marriage ended and this was, I believe, to have a significant impact on the work with James.

Initial sessions

At the beginning I saw James in the office and we discussed the impending transfer to the ILP, and my idea for him to have access to his files. I put it to him that he had been 'looked after' and had had contact with social workers for most of his life and sometimes young people forget how they ended up in the care system, or are confused about events in their lives. James agreed to this idea and we met a fortnight later in the office.

James arrived for the next session as arranged, which I was relieved at, as I knew that the work was inevitably going to bring up painful memories and feelings for him. We talked about where to start. I wanted James to have some choice, and we looked at different distinct phases in his life. During the course of our conversation, it became quite clear to me that he could remember a lot about earlier events – his period in foster care in Kent, being sexually abused, his mother's violent partners – going back to when he was about six years old. This made it difficult for me to know where to start, because the list appeared to represent so many difficult and painful events in James' life.

In the end, with my help he chose the 18-month period when he was in Kent in foster care some six years earlier. James read some reports from that period, which was characterised by (i) he left boarding school and moved out of London; (ii) he had two disrupted placements. James did not make a lot of comments, but I did want to ask him why he felt the placements had broken down and he told me that he was too far out of London (approximately 40 miles) and too far away from his mother, and he only saw her once a month. I acknowledged with him that in hindsight we should have listened to him more at the time, because I remember he had said repeatedly that he wanted to be back in London. I ended by asking him if he had any photos of his carers from this period. He told me he had none, and we agreed I would try to get some. He could add these to his life story book.

Before the next session, James 'phoned me up and said he did not want to continue with the work and we spoke briefly on the 'phone about the reasons. He told me that his mother did not like it. I suggested that he come into the office as arranged so that we could talk about it (James was at home, so staying close to the office).

James arrived for the appointment and we discussed his reservations about carrying on with the work. What emerged was that, at first, he stuck to his story that his mother did not like him doing it; but more importantly he said he did not want to "bring up all that old stuff – it was too painful". I empathised with his feelings but felt unsure what to do. I knew from our earlier discussions that James had not blocked off completely painful events. I was also aware that I had stirred up memories and feelings from many years ago.

Before the meeting I knew that there was going to be some resistance to carrying on the work and I did not know how far to push James into continuing with the work. I felt as a 17-year-old he had to have a choice in the matter. I put it to him, therefore, that he might find it helpful if I put in writing for him a summary of his life in care, and how I had perceived he had developed over the years. He agreed to this, which did not surprise me, but I thought, what a task I've given myself!

After this meeting, obviously the original focus had shifted, and I found it difficult to keep to regular appointments because of annual leave and course commitments. The transfer meeting to the ILP did not take place as arranged. I had arranged it during a week when I was to be off work, but I promised to come in for it because of its importance. However, I completely forgot about the date until I arrived back from leave. The ILP worker was understandably angry, and I was very disappointed that I had let James down, as he had turned up for the meeting.

Transfer to ILP

For the next two months the time-scales began to drift to a serious extent in terms of the transfer to the ILP, as I did not speak to the ILP worker. On reflection, this was an indication of my ambivalence about ending my work with James and reflecting his feelings. I did meet up with James and his mother and they both expressed a wish that James remain in care beyond his 18th birthday, which seemed to be another indicator of James' resistance to ending our relationship.

My response was to say to James and his mother that I thought it probably was not possible, but at the same time I suggested that it could be discussed at his statutory review. At his review there was a full discussion, but it was made clear by my manager that it was probably not possible for James to stay with his foster carer for very long past his 18th birthday. Reflecting my lack of contact with the ILP, the worker did not turn up, even though she had been invited.

After returning from annual leave, I was surprised to find a date had been set for the following day with the ILP for the transfer meeting. Without thinking, I agreed to go ahead and 'phoned up James, who was agreeable to the date and time. Not surprisingly, James did not turn up for the meeting and it went ahead in his absence, with myself formally agreeing to transfer the files in the first week of the following month. I was concerned that James had not been involved in the discussion, so I got the ILP social worker to agree to a meeting with myself and James at my office the following week.

Between that date and the proposed meeting, I drafted the letter which I had promised to do, on my perception of significant events in his life. During the course of this piece of work, which contained many events for James around separation and loss, unexpectedly enormous emotional feelings were triggered off about the end of my marriage, and the realisation that I had known James nearly as long as my wife.

The following week James did arrive for the meeting and just prior to it the ILP worker 'phoned to say that she would be a few minutes late. Unfortunately she was half an hour late, so James and I got into a discussion about his moving on. He expressed extremely ambivalent feelings about moving on, saying the ILP were "rubbish, a bunch of idiots – they never contact me". In this exchange, I experienced strong feelings of counter-transference. I could not acknowledge with James his feelings of loss or that I would miss him too, because our meeting had triggered again my own loss.

Fortunately the ILP worker arrived and I felt I was being rescued by her. I explained to her what we had been discussing and she was able to acknowledge much better than I could James' feelings and fears about moving on. She reassured James that he would not have to make an instant decision about living in his own flat, and that there were stages to full independence; that he did not have to make definite decisions when his care order ended, although he would be expected to move from his foster carer.

I hoped that her contribution had helped James and at the end we were able to discuss final visits; arrangements were made to show James the letter I had written for him. After the meeting, I went outside and walked around the building to let go of the emotions I had been containing. I had gone into the office but there was nobody appropriate around to talk to as it was lunchtime and the summer holiday period.

Ending the work

It was only after this meeting that I consciously realised that over the preceding months I had been mirroring James' ambivalence in not ending the work because I was still dealing with the issues around the end of my marriage. The ending of my work with James had become enmeshed in the ending of my marriage, so I was not able to deal with James' feelings of loss and the work had drifted on. Just as I was not able to control my emotions at this time, the usual control that I felt I exerted over the case went adrift as well. I was determined, however, to face the feelings of loss which I was experiencing and to try and see through ending the work with James as soon as possible.

I did not keep to the deadline for transferring the files because I had to discuss with my supervisor on his return from leave the feelings this work had evoked in me before I felt I could 'end' it in a more appropriate manner. I also re-read writings by Jewett (1984) and Adcock et al (1988), which helped me re-focus on the ending of the work. A few weeks went by before I arranged to meet James and again he did not turn up for the appointment. After a number of attempts to contact him, I eventually saw him at his mother's home.

At this meeting, my emotions still felt fragile. I tried to explore with him why he had been avoiding me, but he simply focused on problems he was having with Mrs Appleby, his foster carer, which I acknowledged needed discussing, but I suggested he needed to talk to his social worker at the ILP and I would tell her that he had raised the issues with me. I did not at this stage want to be drawn into further meetings as another deadline for transfer had passed, and I did not want my involvement to drift on much longer.

I shared with him the letter I had written which he skimmed through without much comment, but he surprised me when he said that he had read a lot of the information about his early years from the court affidavits I had written in connection with the wardship proceedings seven years earlier. I laughed and realised children and young people know a lot more than we think.

We discussed arrangements for our final meeting. James and I had talked about it before and I had given him some choice in what he wanted to do and whom he wanted to bring along. He told me that he would like to go for a meal with myself and his mother. We arranged this for the following week.

We met as arranged for our meal in a restaurant. Right up to the last minute I did not know (i) whether they would turn up; or (ii) whether I could contain my feelings of sadness. James did turn up and on meeting he told me that he had got a new job in Hertfordshire (near where his foster carer had moved), working shifts on a production line in a factory. I congratulated him and felt this was good news on our last meeting together, and it gave me a sense of satisfaction that he had managed to go out and find a job. I was thankful that James and his mother did turn up and we had a good meal and an enjoyable evening. We were able to talk a little about the past and laugh about some experiences, which at the time had not been amusing for me.

I was also able to express to James for the first time my own feelings that I would miss him and how much I had enjoyed working with James and his mother. I was able to tell James I had never worked with a young person so long before, and that I hoped he would call into the office and let me know how he was getting on. James did not say anything in particular; his mother thanked me for my comments. I felt relieved that at last I had been able to acknowledge with him my feelings about the ending. We said our goodbyes and as we went our separate ways I felt a sense of relief that we had had an enjoyable evening, and I wondered when I might see James or his mother again in the office.

Evaluation

This was undoubtedly the most painful and difficult piece of work I have undertaken. At one stage I wondered whether the ending would ever come. Looking back, with the benefit of hindsight, I found myself not only grieving over the end of my relationship with James, but the end of my marriage as well. As a result, I could not deal with James' feelings of sadness, anger, loss and the issue of avoidance.

I identified this piece of work early in the Goldsmiths course because I felt that having worked with James I wanted to have a 'good' ending and I hoped that by reading around the subject of endings I could produce a good piece of focused work. Having completed the work I feel dissatisfied that it took so long. I know that organisationally I became very sloppy because of my own resistance to ending the work. I should have made more effort to speak to James' mother at the beginning about his access to files, as she admitted to me it brought up painful memories for her. I should also have kept in closer touch with his foster carer.

Reflecting on the initial period, I can see that my failure to chase the ILP about rearranging the transfer meeting reflected not only my ambivalence about ending the relationship, but a belief echoed by Stein and Carey (1986) that, given the breakdown rates for young people in care, a more flexible approach should be taken to policies on leaving care. While I recognise that the ILP does provide support after young people leave care, and there is provision in Section 24 of the Children Act (1989), I question the rigid policies on young people leaving their foster placement around their 18th birthday.

This possibility was explored at James' statutory review but we were told it was not possible. As I write this, I still do not know whether I am over-identifying with James because, of course, in his case he would simply return home to his mother's flat and I have already expressed my fears about that situation. What we do know is that leaving home is difficult for any young person, but young people leaving care, I believe, are more vulnerable generally because of their previous life experiences.

With regard to the emotions evoked during the course of the work, although they have been difficult to handle, it has been a tremendous learning experience in terms of getting me in touch with feelings around separation and loss. I am also aware that in attempting to work with James in this way, I was taking a very different approach to my past work with him. I am disappointed that James and I were not able to carry on looking at the past, and I am still left wondering what he has done with all those painful feelings.

I wonder whether gender was an issue for James. I know that it is only in the recent past, as our relationship improved, that I have been able to discuss feelings with him, but with difficulty. In the past his main experience of talking about feelings has been with women, and my approach has been very task-centred. With regard to the letter I wrote for James, I feel very pleased with it and I hope in the long term that it achieves the aim I identified earlier from Triseliotis (1983), that James would be perceived by others as a worthwhile person.

Finally, although I feel a lot of dissatisfaction with my social work practice in this piece of work, I was pleased that we were able to have an ending. I thought it was particularly symbolic that James chose to invite his mother along for the meal, and it gave me a tremendous sense of satisfaction that, having removed James some seven years earlier from his mother, we were all sitting around the table together at the end.

In the course of the meal, James talked about his extended family and visits to them in the Isle of Man. For me it felt like James had been reintegrated as far as possible back into his family, except for his father, who had left when he was two years old. I was so pleased that on our last meeting together James had found himself employment. This, I hope, will be the beginning for him in attempting to achieve economic independence, which is important for adolescents in their attempts to make the transition to adulthood.

Eve:
From victim to healthy survivor?

Mary Cody

Purpose of the intervention

Eve, aged 13 years, was placed for adoption three years ago with her half sibling Simon, aged 11 years. Her parents have become increasingly concerned about Eve's unpredictable mood swings. She is verbally and physically abusive and recently there has been a pattern of running away. Eve is a white British girl placed in a family who reflect her racial and cultural origins. The family contacted their local social services department and together they have agreed the need for work with the family and the need for direct work with Eve.

As a voluntary adoption agency we have been approached to undertake the direct work. The initial contract is to have six sessions with Eve, to help her get in touch with how she is feeling about herself in order to plan appropriate intervention. Winnicott (1984) says "the immediate purpose of communication is to get in touch with children's real selves, what they are feeling about themselves and their lives". It was important to recognise at the outset that where Eve was the focus of concern the family did have a more systemic perspective and were motivated to engage in exploring their part in the current dynamic.

Theoretical and experiential Influences

Having read Eve's history, I thought that insights from attachment theory could illuminate some of the current concerns. John Bowlby's (1980) work highlights the central significance of attachment for healthy emotional and psychological development. Bowlby uses the concept of inner working models to describe how interactions with significant figures are internalised and carried into subsequent relationships and experiences. Knowledge and understanding of the internal representational aspects of attachment was important in connecting Eve's behaviour to her feelings and her past experiences.

Awareness not only of the roots of attachment theory in Bowlby's work, but also of the growing points in the work of Mary Main (1991) was necessary in developing a sense of hope. Much of Mary Main's work focuses on the ability to make sense of past experiences, as a factor mitigating their influence in current relationships. This is similar to Barbara Dockar-Drysdale's (1968) notion of 'conceptualisation' of early experiences, as a necessary stage in getting in control of them and removing some of their power.

Understanding the process whereby internal working models of the 'self' form alongside representations of attachment figures, helped in thinking about Eve's lack of any real sense of worth or self-esteem. This conceptual framework was very valuable in developing insight around how these models could be now ordering and informing Eve's experiences, rather than current experiences having any real impact on her 'inner working models'.

David Howe's (1995) work was useful in providing a conceptual framework within which to explore Eve's current pattern of attachments, particularly around ambivalent and resistant behaviours. This work also provided me with insight into the nature and development of defence mechanisms. Goodrich et al's (1990) work with adopted adolescents helped to further tune my antennae to the role of defences such as denial, splitting and projective identification in my contact with Eve. While I was very aware of the presence of Eve's well developed defence system, I felt a degree of anxiety and inexperience in interpreting the transference. This highlighted the importance of supervision/ consultation in exploring and making sense of what was happening within my relationship with Eve, in recognising and understanding symbolic levels of communication.

In approaching my work with Eve I was really influenced by the feelings evoked while reviewing her history. It seemed in so many ways that Eve had spent the first seven years of her life crying out to be heard. The phrase 'it takes two to tell the truth: one to say it and another to hear it' kept echoing inside me. Her current behaviour was speaking volumes and I hoped that by creating some space to listen she might feel empowered and begin to take back some control over her life.

Process of the work

Case records

In reviewing the process of the work I will start at the beginning, with Eve's history. Reviewing Eve's case records was a very harrowing and powerful exercise. From the lengthy and detailed narratives, seven years of almost continuous rejection, neglect, physical and sexual abuse emerged. This was Eve's 'story' and what really hit me was that it had taken so long to validate what was happening, seven years to say, yes, something terrible is happening to this child and it must stop.

In reviewing the file I began to formulate ideas and hypotheses about the current concerns which I would explore further in the direct work. The stage was set before Eve was born in terms of attachment being a key concern. Joan, her birth mother, had a long history of poor attachments and alcohol abuse. Heavy drinking throughout her pregnancy resulted in concerns about intrauterine growth retardation and microcephaly in relation to Eve. Poor developmental progress and failure to thrive were quickly added to the list. By the age of three months family centre staff were noting how her mother's partner 'smacked' her on the bottom.

I thought that Eve's needs had been so unmet, so early in life, that she really had no opportunity to get her emotional 'bank account' in credit. She had no reserves to draw on when the going got tough. Bowlby's work explores the infant's intrinsic need for stable and reliable attachments as a foundation for mental health. Eve's perception of the world as laid down during her early years must be of an unpredictable and hurtful place. How could she have accomplished the primary psychological task of developing trust in others?

While the case records helped me identify where Eve's needs had not been met, I was also alerted to the feelings precipitated in Eve by her experiences and had some clues as to how she had coped with stress in the past. Her foster carers comment that "Eve takes everything as such a personal attack: nothing is ever enough for her", heightened my awareness of her internal representations of relationships.

Before meeting with Eve I met with her parents. I wanted to explain what I would be doing with Eve and get them alongside us:

> Direct work cannot be successfully done in a vacuum. It is something
> that needs to be planned and co-ordinated … in co-operation with

other significant adults in the child's life. (Aldgate and Simmonds, 1988, p 8)

We would review the work after six sessions and would share some of the feelings after each session.

Direct work sessions

During my first meeting with Eve we negotiated a contract during a walk round a local lake. The walk was Eve's suggestion and, I thought, placed us 'alongside' each other rather than 'eyeball to eyeball'. Eve agreed that life at home was very unhappy at times and that space for her to think about what was happening might help. She said "Nobody ever listens to me" and allowed me to say that this was what I wanted to do. We set some boundaries around the sessions and around sharing information. When we returned home Eve plotted our six sessions on the calendar and supervised their insertion in my diary. Being reliable and consistent was going to be so important.

During the direct work with Eve a number of incidents presented themselves to be understood (see interview abstracts). They were interrelated and real enactments of where Eve's 'internal working models' were functioning, in a way that made them a real pervasive and destructive influence on her thoughts, feelings and actions. Vera Fahlberg (1994) speaks of early unmet needs coming back to haunt adolescents and this seemed to be happening here. During one session with Eve she did a 'sculpt' of her family with some play people. She placed herself on the edge of the family with Simon between her parents some distance apart. In exploring this further with questions around whether this was how Eve wanted it and what she would change for it to be different, she responded with "It's always been like this; you just get used to it".

Box 1: Abstract from second session with Eve

Mum and Eve had a row around whether Eve could be left alone in the house while mum went to work for a couple of hours. The row escalated with Eve becoming very abusive. Mum went to work leaving Eve alone, and shortly had a 'phone call from the police who had been called to the house by neighbours.

I arrived as the police were leaving, mum in tears and Eve in her room screaming and banging. I spent a little time with mum hearing her story of treading on eggshells with Eve, tripping over landmines she could not see, and feeling quite unsupported at times by her husband and wider family.

When I went upstairs Eve had quietened though I could hear real sobbing. When I knocked and opened the door Eve was lying curled in a tight ball on the floor with her arms around her head. The room was a mess. It took some time for Eve to become calm and we did some breathing and relaxing exercises together. When she could speak she kept repeating in a baby voice "she left me". It was some time before Eve could put into words what had happened but her feelings and perception of being abandoned and rejected were there in all her body language. I was reminded of the work done by Bessel van der Kolk around trauma. He offers the view that "victims of trauma respond to contemporary stimuli as if the trauma returned. This interferes with their ability to make calm and rational assessments. Extreme responses ensue."

It certainly seemed as if this current event had tapped into a deep well of feelings and that Eve was having real difficulty in distinguishing what 'was' from what 'is'. Her chaos and confusion was exposed and felt very raw. With Eve's agreement mum joined us and with support Eve was able to ask for, and allowed herself to be held, by her mum. I could see the lack of trust in Eve's stiffness. It was almost impossible for her to construe her mum as a reliable person. I focused on affirming their reciprocal feelings of confusion while offering some tentative interpretations of what had happened. I thought Eve's mum was able to hear, but for Eve such insight was a long way off.

Box 2: Abstract from fourth session with Eve

Eve's mum met me at the door in a state of agitated distress. She led me into the sitting room where Eve was lying on the sofa covered in blood. Her eye was badly cut, her nose bleeding and some of her hair pulled out. She and another girl had been involved in a fight in the classroom in the last lesson. Eve was clinging to her mum and repeating her name. She became quite agitated when her mum went to get some water to clean her up. I noticed that both of Eve's hands and part of her forearms were covered in the most intricate patterns drawn in ink.

As Eve was eventually able to put the day into some sort of order a picture emerged of a young person quite removed from the work of the classroom. Her time was not spent attending to the lesson but rather in drawing patterns on her hands. Was this a way of blocking out feelings, especially bad feelings, of worthlessness and incompetence? It only took one taunt from this girl to unleash a torrent of rage from Eve. Eve was able to talk about how she felt prior to the incident and if one word sums up her feelings it would have to be 'persecuted'. Eve spoke of how it had "always been like this" and "you get used to it". At one level she could see that her response was so extreme and she was able to connect her reaction to her feelings.

Eve was able to go on to name other occasions when she had been enraged by what were really minor annoyances including a recent occasion when she had hit her mum. It seemed incidents were occurring all the time where Eve was so ready to misperceive, misconstrue and misinterpret what was happening. Eve was able to acknowledge how hurts in the here and now seemed to lead to a re-living of all the hurts of the past, yet the memory of these hurts was sitting in a part of Eve that had no words but perceptions and feelings that were so easily triggered.

She then went on to create her foster family and her birth family in a similar pattern, with Simon located between the adults and herself on the periphery. Her very ambivalent feelings found some expression in exploring this: the very hard "I don't need them, I don't care" alongside envy and jealousy. This session really preoccupied me and I felt quite depressed afterwards. I found this hard to explain as I thought Eve had confirmed my view of what was happening in the family or at least how she might be experiencing it. It was only in supervision that I was able to use my feelings to get in touch with the transference and the very real sense of despair and hopelessness that Eve was projecting in exploring repeated experiences of family life.

Story stems

Eve's perceptions of life were illuminated further during a session when we worked with some narrative story stems (Buchsbaum et al, 1992). Her very clear expectation that adults would not help when children were hurt emerged, as did her experience that aggression should and would form a part of any solution to a dilemma. I began one story stem with Eve cooking in the kitchen with mum. Eve is warned about the danger of being so close to the hot plate; she then gets burned. Eve continued the story with a very punitive, aggressive response from mum, accompanied by much swearing. Eve then went off on her own to treat her burn.

Throughout this and some other story stems Eve conveyed a real sense of victimisation, alongside anger and aggression. Often the stories disintegrated into chaos and incoherence once aggression set in. A further related theme which emerged in my contact and which I had a number of opportunities to observe was Eve's inability to recognise 'good experiences'. If she did experience any positive feelings they were fleeting and certainly she had no way of storing them. She literally shrugged off any positive strokes that came her way.

This was highlighted for me on hearing Eve's mum's account of her horseriding skills and care of the horse as a stable hand. She seemed to respond to praise, encouragement and support as if what she was hearing was criticism. It was so easy for her to discount the plusses that came her way, whereas the slightest criticism was felt like a stab wound. Her internal model of herself as unlovable and undeserving of good things seemed immune to the healing impact of nurturing experiences.

The six sessions ended as pre-planned with the next stage being to share perceptions of 'what might be wrong' and to look at possible ways forward in terms of intervention.

Analysis and evaluation of the work

The purpose of this piece of work was to reach an understanding of how Eve was feeling about herself and her world. There were three interrelated routes to greater understanding of Eve's perceptual world. I started with the belief that understanding her history of attachments and developmental experiences could help me in making sense of some the current concerns. Reviewing her file heightened my awareness of the importance of preparation.

This first glimpse into Eve's world not only helped me develop ideas and hypotheses which I could later explore but also helped to prepare me for the emotional impact of the work. From the records I formed some possible pictures of Eve's internal representations of attachment relationships and of herself. Those pictures were informed not only by the facts but underpinned by theoretical and experiential influences.

In direct contact with Eve, both through live incidents which shouted out to be understood and worked with, and more structured directed sessions, the clarity and vividness of her world emerged. Through direct observation of her interactions, especially with her mum, and her narrative accounts of day-to-day life, I saw not only how her 'working models' were impacting on her daily life but also how resistant to change they were. Alongside this the impact of past traumatic experiences was so clear, as was her dissociation. While her records contained a catalogue of drunken brawls with police intervention, Eve did not "know my mum drank". These traumatic memories are laid down in a part of Eve that has no words.

Through this piece of work my primary aim was to make space to listen, to affirm rather than interpret. I wanted Eve to feel understood and endeavoured to convey this to her. In terms of the work informing the questions 'where now' and 'what next', a number of things are clear. Eve needs the opportunity to reappraise and reconstruct the past. There will be great resistance to this and it can only happen at her pace. It will take a long time for her to own and understand the pieces of her life. She needs to be empowered with permission and support to do this work.

This piece of work has been so full of new learning for me. Not having worked with an adolescent before I was quite apprehensive and concerned that Eve would be bearing the cost of my learning. There were times when I found the work very absorbing and preoccupying and I became quite aware of the need to maintain healthy functioning boundaries. Supervision was essential in enabling this and in helping me unravel and process the myriad of feelings being evoked. I have been very torn between feeling 'time is of the essence', wanting to call in 'a team of specialists', and recognising that Eve and her family have the beginnings of a trusting relationship and this work cannot be hurried. It needs time, space and commitment and containment. I am planning to take the work further and endeavouring to secure more specialist consultation in undertaking this.

This piece of work highlighted for me the long-term and pervasive legacy of childhood trauma. It made me think again about the preparation and support of all families, birth families, foster and adoptive families who care for these young people and who undertake so much of the reparenting work. The resource implications must not be forgotten, nor minimised as such documents as past drafts of the Adoption Bill sought to do, in seeing the provision of post–adoption services as 'cost-neutral'. The work involved in enabling a young person like Eve to become less of a victim and more of a healthy survivor needs commitment at every level, from the individual worker through to the legislature.

Amos and Christopher:
Working towards care proceedings

Michael O'Dempsey

Position at the outset

Amos (age 7) and Christopher (age 8) are brothers who were subject to interim care orders and living in foster care. They have a younger brother, John (age 2), who was living with their mother. They are of mixed race. Their mother is Asian Muslim and their father is white European. Their parents had separated and their father was seeking a residence order (see genogram, Figure 1).

The parental relationship was characterised by domestic violence, arguments, the racial abuse of the mother by the father, denial of contact with their father and the constant denigration of each parent by the other. Due to this the children's names were included on the child protection register under the category of emotional abuse, and care programmes were underway.

Assessment: children's situation

The children were experiencing a major 'psychosocial' change due to their parents' divorce. Bohannen (1971) describes children of divorcing parents as experiencing a number of processes including that of the 'psychic divorce', in which children mourn the loss of their old family before they can adjust to their new situation. Even in the best managed divorces that is a very difficult process. Many additional factors existed within this family system, making this process more difficult. These boys had also been separated from their mother three times within six months.

Mothers who have experienced domestic violence describe their children as feeling sad and lacking self-esteem, being protective towards their mother and feeling guilty. The children displayed confusion and emotional turmoil (NCH Action for Children, 1994). Carrol (1994) states "Children who witness aggressive outbursts may be traumatised by the violent episodes themselves".

Figure 1: Genogram

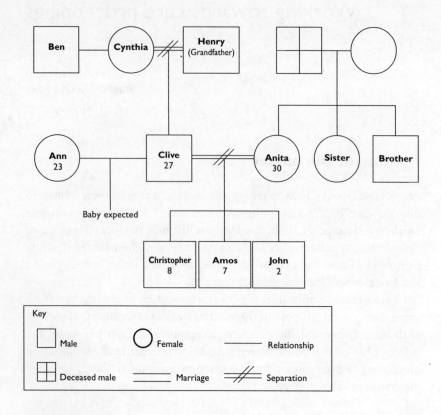

I became aware of the impact of domestic violence on the children when Amos described witnessing his father banging his mother's head against a wall. Amos feared that her "head would crack". Amos generally presents as outgoing and confident but as he described this incident he appeared quiet, sad, deflated and frightened. Later, while in foster care, he again mentioned this violence as if he had witnessed it recently. Amos said that he wanted to return to live with his mother to stop his parents fighting.

Christopher is less confident than Amos, has few friends and frequently appears sad and withdrawn. He was more overtly concerned for his mother's health and happiness and indicated that he felt responsible for her. For example, he said "If mum isn't well enough to look after us, we would go home and look after her". Christopher confided to me that he believed that they were in care because they had made their parents argue.

Both Amos and Christopher experienced attachment difficulties with their mother (Iwaniec, 1995) and feared for her safety, health and happiness. When she was upset Christopher was reluctant to leave her even though he was often the focus of her anger and frustration at these times. Both children stated that they wished to return to their mother.

Amos and Christopher were finding it difficult to make sense of their situation and their uncertain future. In an attempt to accommodate himself to this uncertainty Christopher blamed himself for being in care. Amos made a plan for each of them to spend a day alone with their mother in rotation and wished to divide his time between his parents. I was unable to offer the children any certainties as I could not prejudge the Court's decision.

The children's immediate needs

The children experienced great uncertainty as they were living away from home, and were caught between warring parents. It was possible that the Court might send them to live with their father or even strangers. They needed support in making sense of their situation and in addressing their feelings of responsibility regarding this and their own separation from their mother.

Being in foster care protected the children from witnessing further violence and argument between their parents. However, they remained vulnerable to their parents' mutual criticism during contact. Amos in particular experienced pressure from his father, who told him to say that he wanted to live with him.

Negotiation with colleagues and others

Direct work

I arranged with the children and their foster carer that I would visit on Monday evenings and we would use their room for the sessions. This was agreed with their parents at Court and at a Child in Care Review.

Supervision

My supervisor had recently left to take up a new post and a new supervisor was appointed shortly before the final hearing. In the interim, I was supervised by an independent social worker. I consulted with my practice coordinator and Goldsmiths College regarding a suitable approach to the direct work. My team manager agreed that I should receive specialist supervision from a child psychotherapist for this direct work. This became available just before the Court hearing, by which time the children had returned to their mother's care.

Guardian ad litem

The children quickly formed a trusting relationship with their guardian *ad litem* and they understood that she would tell the judge their wishes. However, she became ill and retired from the case. The children then had to make a relationship with a new guardian who also agreed with and supported my planned direct work with the children.

Foster carers

During the children's placement their foster carers separated. This potentially left them re-experiencing the distress they had endured around their parents' separation. It could have reinforced their 'phantasy' (Segal, 1985) that they caused their carers to separate. It was a tribute to the foster carer that the boys were to continue living with her without apparently experiencing these feelings. The foster carer was, in turn, well supported by her link worker, with whom I also liaised.

Influences which have shaped my intervention

Choice of intervention

It was impossible to work with the family as a whole as the parents' mutual hostility rendered them unable to participate simultaneously. Had this been attempted the children would be at risk of witnessing further abusive and violent arguments. It was unlikely that individual work with their father would be productive as he had dismissed previous attempts to engage him. Their mother was supported by a family centre social worker in addressing her experiences of loss and its impact on her ability to care for the children.

Therefore I hoped to help the children through an open-ended programme of direct work aimed at exploring with them their experiences prior to accommodation and their wishes and feelings. I hoped to help them recognise that they were not responsible for their parents' separation or their being 'in care'.

The children's developmental stages

Erikson's model of identity development (Open University, 1990) was invaluable in planning my work. This describes children's identities as developing through stages at which particular aspects of identity become the focus of development and are vulnerable to damage. These stages each contain an essential dilemma, the successful resolution of which enables the child to form the basis for later stages of identity development.

Christopher (age 8) and Amos (age 7) were in their 'schooldays' (latency) period when children must resolve the dilemma between task identification and a sense of futility. Latency is usually considered a calmer period compared to the turmoil of early childhood. Through their early troubled years Amos and Christopher had not had an opportunity to resolve the earlier stages of identity development satisfactorily.

Throughout these sessions my work with the children was greatly influenced by their constantly changing circumstances and the influence of the children's father, who expressed a negative attitude towards my work, thereby undermining my attempts to help them.

Protecting the children from further exposure to arguments between their parents and witnessing further violence

During the course of my work the children were successfully reunited with their mother. The children continued to have contact with their father, who collected and returned them from their mother's home. This presented a risk of their witnessing further arguments and abuse. To avoid this I negotiated that a childminder act as a go-between.

Goals and working methods chosen

Goals

- To enable Christopher and Amos to express their wishes and feelings in order to present these in my report to the Court and to communicate these to their parents.
- To allow them to talk about their experiences of being caught between their parents and the pressure that this put them under.
- To support them through a period of great uncertainty and their feelings of vulnerability from having been separated from their mother.

- To help them to resolve their inappropriate feelings of responsibility for their parents' separation and being taken into care.
- To help them to resolve their feelings of distress from having witnessed domestic violence.

Methods

- I visited Amos and Christopher weekly at their foster carer's home at the same time each week for 40 minutes.
- I used several techniques in helping them to express themselves, such as:
  - ‣ techniques for enabling them to externalise their feelings through a third object (Redgrave, 1987). This 'barrier breaking' technique enabled the children to express themselves without restricting them to their language development.
  - ‣ I found sociograms (Redgrave, 1987) and drawings useful aids in helping them to describe family relationships and as triggers to discussion.
  - ‣ On occasion the children or I would write down their stories or opinions. This helped us to focus on our discussion and signalled that their views were important.
  - ‣ I used objects such as lego, toy people and toy cars to engage the children in symbolic play (Cattenach, 1994). This technique became especially useful in the latter phase of my work in helping Christopher to express his secret wishes that he has been unable to tell his mother. In symbolic play he was able to acknowledge his secret wish that his parents would reunite and subsequently he was able to tell his mother.
  - ‣ I found some awareness of psychodynamic concepts (Jacobs, 1988) helpful in acknowledging my response to the material the children presented to me.

Establishing a therapeutic environment

When I visited on Monday evenings we used the children's room to avoid constant interruptions by the foster carers' children. Amos and Christopher share a history and have been each other's only constant relationship and I believed that they would find each other's presence supportive. I planned to allow them as much freedom of expression as possible in the sessions. I took a large pad of paper and felt pens to each session.

In the first session I explained why I was seeing them and that I would be telling the judge what they wanted to happen and also what I thought was best for them. We agreed some rules: the children suggested a rule that they would not hit each other in the sessions. Each session began with sharing news and later I helped them express and discuss their concerns. We had eight sessions before and six after they returned to their mother.

Addressing issues of discrimination

The issue of race is very complex in this family. It may be noted that the children's family home showed no obvious influence of their mother's Asian upbringing. Indeed she prides herself that she could pass as Italian. This suggested that she internalised the effects of societal racism which resulted in a 'spoiled identity' (Goffman, 1968) and the denial of her own racial identity and that of her children. The racism she experienced in her marriage had reinforced this. The children's white British foster carer's life-style reflected that of their own family but did not offer a model which affirmed their mixed parentage identity (Small, 1989). I attempted to reinforce a positive self-image in the children.

The issue of racial identity is highlighted by a family myth which split the children along the lines of their appearance. This stated that Christopher, who looked Asian, was made by their mother; whereas Amos, who looked white, had been made by their father. This placed Amos in a difficult position as he identified himself with his father whom he said he hated. Their brother John was said to have been made by both parents. This mirrored societal issues of racial identity within the family. Their racial identity and self-esteem had been further damaged through witnessing the racial abuse of their mother by their father.

Through discussion with a consultant on race at Goldsmiths College I came to understand that while their mother was in denial of her own racial identity, one could not expect her to be able to provide a positive attitude towards her children's emerging racial identity. Therefore it was likely that they would need support with this in the future.

In common with the father, I am a white male and the children had witnessed their white father's racial and physical abuse of their Asian mother. I was aware that this might reinforce the patriarchal model they had experienced within their family (Dominelli, 1988). I sensed pressure from their father to collude with him in criticising their mother;

when he realised that I would not collude he began criticising me to the children.

Process

The session prior to reunification with their mother

During the initial sessions I found the children's demands for attention overwhelming. They fought continuously. I was unable to focus my attention on either child as the other would distract me. I felt that this arose from their own individual needy feelings. Therefore I arranged to see them both together for a few minutes at the start and end of each session, but would see them separately during the session.

Amos was troubled at the prospect of telling me about his feelings and he adopted a persona when he was alone with me in the first session. He called himself 'Mr Banana Head'. To engage with Amos I had first to engage with 'Mr Banana Head', who voiced a very low opinion of Amos. It was only after I said that I liked Amos and thought he was a good boy that 'Mr Banana Head' left the room to change (literally his clothes) and Amos came to speak with me. I was initially very concerned that Amos was finding his situation so distressing that he had split into another personality in order to cope (Jacobs, 1988). This has not reoccurred.

Following sessions

Over the following sessions several themes emerged.

Issues of racial identity and self-esteem

Christopher suffered low self-esteem and 'spoiled identity'. When he drew me a picture/sociogram of his family, he drew a segmented wheel-like image. He drew mother, father, brothers, a goblin (who featured in a story he told earlier in the session) and myself. Christopher said "Shall I show you who I love?" He then drove a toy car around the wheel, tracing its journey with a pen. The trail ended with his mother.

Then he said "Shall I show you who I hate?" Christopher drove the car around the map again and I expected him to stop the car by me (earlier he had been angry with me). Christopher stopped the car at his own picture. I asked Christopher why he hated himself. Christopher said that he did not like his name or his skin and did not like himself. I asked him what he would like to be called and he said Michael (a name

I share with his mother's boyfriend). My supervisor suggested that Christopher may have attached his low self-esteem and feelings of detachment to the obvious physical differences between himself and his brother.

For Amos, his racial identity was more complex as the family myth identified him with his father. Amos had expressed a negative view of his family and was distressed due to pressure from his father.

Loss and abandonment

The early sessions frequently involved the children expressing feelings of loss and abandonment. This was evident in Amos' sociograms in which all the important people in his life are on the outside inch of the paper with nothing at its centre. I was surprised by this and repeated the exercise in a later session. Amos drew a remarkably similar map. I asked him who would come to help him if he needed help. Amos initially said his gang would help him but later revealed that he had no gang and he didn't believe his parents would help him.

In the ensuing silence I felt a great sadness, which I took to be a transference of Amos' sadness (Jacobs, 1988). To acknowledge this I said "That sounds very sad". Amos left the room. Later I found him and sensing his despair I said that I would come to help him. I now recognise that I may have been responding to my own feelings of helplessness in the face of his despair but this illustrates a conflict of roles. In my role as his social worker I would come to help him, but in a purely psychodynamic counselling relationship my promise may be seen as blurring my role.

Christopher's feelings of abandonment were communicated most clearly through his stories and drawings. During one session he drew a picture of himself falling off a mountain. In his accompanying story he fell off a mountain and shouted 'help'. He then landed on a snow flake and a burglar picked him up and ate him. When he uttered these words Christopher immediately changed the story. In his new and less overwhelming version his mother found him on the snow flake and took him home and I came to help her look after him.

Assessing the children's wishes

Ultimately both children were able to give me clear and consistent messages about their wishes. Christopher had always been very clear that he wanted to live with his mother. In a session with Amos I sensed his great anxiety that he would be sent to live with his father. I drew two figures, one representing his mother and the other his father. Amos had indicated that he felt emotionally torn by his parents. We tore a figure which represented Amos and I said "I think that's what it feels like for you". Amos didn't speak and then he took a pen and wrote on the piece of his image which went to his mother "I want to live with mum". Then on the piece which went to his father he wrote "I don't want to live with dad", beside which he wrote "I still love you".

The children were reunited with their mother and the Court subsequently granted a residence order to her and a supervision order to the local authority. At this time a child psychotherapist became my supervisor. She advised that I should again work with the children together, since to divide the session may not have allowed sufficient time for themes to be fully explored. While I felt that in theoretical terms my supervisor was correct, I was anxious that I would have difficulty in managing both children together. My supervisor helped me re-explore my feelings of being overwhelmed by the children's needs and suggested that this was a transference of the children's own needy feelings.

Sessions following the children's return home

These sessions also took place on Monday evenings at the local family centre, with which the children were already familiar. During the first of these sessions the children constantly left the room to seek their mother. This made it difficult to focus on our work. By the second session I negotiated that their mother would direct them to return to me if they left the room. However, the children continued to seek her out.

A theme began to emerge in Christopher's response to Amos' play. Amos was putting furniture in a doll's house. When he drew Christopher's attention to this, Christopher threw the furniture through the doll's house window. He displayed similar behaviour in a following session when Amos had rearranged a large play house. I felt that Christopher was disrupting attempts to reconstitute the family. The children at these times would fight.

The second session focused on Christopher's anger towards his father who had smacked him recently. It may be noted that Amos had disclosed the incident. The children's anger was shared by their mother. She declined to attend further sessions. I had anticipated this in supervision and had decided to continue the sessions without her. The children did not leave the room as frequently nor for as long as when she had been near.

During session four, Christopher played with the doll's house. He expressed great hostility towards the baby expected by his father's partner. He said he wanted to kill the baby. Using toys he symbolically placed the baby in a wheel chair and pushed it off the doll's house roof. Later he symbolically buried his father in the sand tray.

Amos modelled his family using multiracial toy people. During this session the boys were especially difficult to manage and I had to restrain them from climbing out of the first floor window at the family centre.

In the fifth session Christopher used lego figures to tell me that he wanted his parents to reunite, and after having said this in the session he was able to tell his mother on his return home.

During the last session Amos disclosed that his mother had struck him with a belt. Amos asked me to speak with her about this. The session was characterised by the children's destructive play. Subsequently their mother acknowledged that she had hit him with a belt. I think that this represented a significant move forward as he trusted me with the expectation that I could contribute to his future protection.

Evaluation of the intervention and feedback

I believe that my intervention with the children was helpful to them as it enabled them to begin to understand that they were not responsible for being in care, nor for their parents fighting and subsequently parting. This was achieved through helping them tell me the story of their parents' separation. I would remind them that I had seen their parents argue even when they were not there. This appeared reassuring to Christopher. It also enabled the children to express their wishes and feelings about their future, which allowed these to be clearly presented to the Court. My regular visiting supported them emotionally through the uncertainty prior to the Court's decision.

I was able to give feedback to their parents. Their father largely dismissed this, but their mother was able to respond to their feelings of abandonment by saying that she would come to help them. The children asked her if she would rescue them from a fire even if it meant her own death. She said she would. The children seemed most reassured by this. When they returned to their mother's care I arranged for her symbolically to reclaim them by collecting them herself from their foster carer.

Subsequent to their return home the children seemed distressed and confused, as they had expected regular contact with their father. He did not maintain his contact, however. Christopher began to articulate his sadness that his parents would not reunite. Amos has expressed interest in his racial identity and has asked his mother about her background. Despite her initial negative response to his curiosity she has begun to accept this.

My work with the children lasted for many months. I found that some of their concerns remained at the conclusion of the sessions. For example Christopher still wished for his parents to reunite. This indicated that he was still attempting to reconcile himself to the process of the 'psychic divorce' of his parents.

What I have learned from this work

Children living through periods of great change are not normally considered to be suitable for psychotherapy. However, the other aspects of my intervention were supportive to them. The children's lives were in a state of great uncertainty, change and readjustment through this period. This contributed to the conflict between my roles. When I first proposed to work with the children together I did not anticipate the demands that they would make of me. A result of this was that I felt overwhelmed by them. I found it extremely difficult to focus on one child without the other disrupting the session.

I was concerned that the children fought more than they did outside the session. Given this I reconsidered my original arrangements and I saw the children separately for the main body of the session. In retrospect I believe that it would have been easier to respond to the children's demands if there had been a co-worker, as we would have been able to respond to their demands for attention and possibly have had them together.

While I was engaged in this work I experienced a great deal of professional change. These changes may be seen as reflecting the changes in the children's own lives. For me these included changes in agency supervisors and my attempting to find and then engage with a specialist supervisor. I had not fully considered the difficulty of reconciling myself to the professional culture of child psychotherapy supervision. Initially this felt de-skilling and I felt that all my early work with the children was of no value.

As our supervision relationship developed my supervisor enabled me to recognise that these transferential feelings may have been similar to the children's feelings towards me during the sessions, characterised by their anger and hostility towards me.

The first phase of my work with the children appeared less prone to difficulties than the sessions at the family centre. This may be because my roles as key worker to the children and as the person doing direct work with them had become most obviously concurrent, now that the children were not protected by living with their foster carer. I was attempting to reconcile these roles and adjust between the child protection worker who was obliged to respond to abusive events in the children's lives, and the role of the person helping them make sense of their experiences. This became especially important when Amos disclosed that his mother had struck him with a belt.

Carol:
Moving to a permanent placement

Stephen Kitchman

Position at the outset

This study relates to a young woman with whom I worked to help her move to a permanent placement in long-term foster care. In order to meet her needs it was necessary to undertake direct work, as well as develop good multiagency communication and future planning for permanency. The agency context was a statutory social services department within a London borough.

I shall initially give brief background history before describing the process and work undertaken, which is illustrated by the theoretical or research basis where appropriate. Later I will describe the outcomes of this work, before offering an evaluation and analysis of my intervention. The reader may assume that all procedures under the Department of Health 'Looked After Children' initiative adopted by the borough have been complied with.

Background

Throughout this study the young woman concerned shall be known as 'Carol'. At the onset of my involvement for the purposes of this work she was 13 years old. Carol was of white British origin and had lived in the borough most of her life. She had no disability although she was statemented for special educational needs, albeit on behavioural grounds. I had been Carol's social worker for approximately seven months, throughout which time she had correspondingly been placed in short-term foster care through a voluntary organisation.

Prior to this, Carol had been looked after under Section 20 of the Children Act (1989) for eight months, following an argument with her mother and a subsequent physical fight. Her mother called the emergency duty team and Carol was placed in emergency foster care late at night. Carol remained looked after and went through a succession of ten placements. Moves on had generally been through short-term placements with the expectation that she would return home, or because the foster carers were unable to cope with her behaviour, which was constantly challenging and verbally abusive. At the onset of this study Carol was in need of a long-term placement.

Carol's family are depicted in the genogram in Figure 1. Both her mother and father had histories of being placed in local authority care, as did all of her siblings. Carol's eldest brother and sister had both been adopted at an early age, due to physical abuse. A care order had been sought unsuccessfully on Robert four years previously, due to suspected sexual abuse by the mother. Carol's sister Jane had been in a 52-week residential school since the age of eight. Both Carol and Jane had alleged sexual abuse by their father and physical abuse by the mother in the year of my involvement. No further action was taken over these allegations due to time-scales, lack of clarity and proof, although the girls had been believed.

Figure 1: Genogram

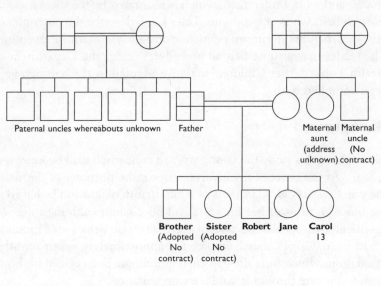

Later this year Carol's father died from a long-standing illness. No contact ensued with Carol's mother, who was extremely negative and rejecting of Carol. There were no positive adult members to support Carol. The only known adult was her mother's brother, with whom there was no contact as he had sexually abused her when she was nine years old; her parents had been supportive to her on this occasion.

Given the above, it was not surprising that Carol's behaviour was extremely turbulent, with frequent mood swings. Carol would swear at her foster carers, particularly the female carer, Ann, and had twice hit her. Following arguments Carol would display entrenched behaviour such as not talking for days. Lack of personal hygiene and an unwillingness to socialise were also concerns of the foster carers, which I believed might be an indication of low self-esteem.

For the seven months that I had been Carol's social worker, much of my input had been reactive through crisis intervention, with child protection allegations against her parents and much advocacy and 'refereeing' work between Carol and her carers to maintain her placement. Indeed, the onset of my involvement had been sparked by an emergency. Fifteen volumes of handwritten files had then been handed to me, of which there was no chronology, current assessment or care plan other than 'to support the placement and continue assessing the situation'. To some extent it felt that I was still following this advice seven months down the line.

Theoretical and experiential influences

Despite continued pressure to take on more casework, I felt it necessary to slow down to take stock of the situation. I aired this in supervision and gained the agreement that Carol needed more focused intervention, to which time could be given. The concerns about Carol's situation were supported by research. Whitaker et al (DoH, 1991b) highlighted the need to have clear and careful aims for successful placements. Similarly, Carol's situation fitted several of the factors associated with placement breakdown postulated by Department of Health (1991b) guidance, namely:

1. Age: breakdowns of all types of placement increase inexorably and often dramatically with increasing age at placement.

2. Previous placement breakdown.

3. The child or young person is ambivalent or opposed to placement.

4. Severe behaviour problems.

5. The child is cut off from all that is familiar by a combination of loss of contact with birth parents, siblings.... (pp 68/9)

It was clear that Carol's placement was at risk of breakdown and the above factors needed to be taken on board and addressed where possible. There seemed to have been little assessment work done to inform the aims, although a wealth of information was available. An appropriate starting point was to attempt an understanding of Carol's history, for as Farmer and Parker (DoH, 1991b) advise us:

Decisions must be placed ... in a context that has an historical dimension. It ought to go without saying that evidence of what has happened in the past provides an important insight into what will happen in the future. (p 69)

I attempted to read as much of the case files as was legible and form a chronology of events and chart Carol's previous placements. I believed that a chronology would be essential, a factor which is documented by many of the child abuse enquiry reports about the need for clear case histories in predicting risk, especially should Carol return home (DoH, 1991a).

Throughout Carol's life there had always been social services involvement. There had been continuous concern over the mother/daughter relationship with, for example, several case references being made to the mother labelling Carol a 'bitch' at the age of one. Family support officers had been involved primarily to support the mother with childcare and also to 'monitor' the situation. There had been ongoing concerns over non-accidental injuries to Carol as a young child but no further action had ensued. File references seemed to indicate that the adult with the most positive view of Carol was her father; sadly he had sexually abused her.

Attachment

The background history raised concerns over Carol's bonding with her mother, with many instances of continual rejection of Carol, as, for example, the health visitor's concerns over physical distancing of Carol. Similarly, I believe apparent lack of bonding from the mother was giving rise to attachment problems for Carol, for as Fahlberg (1994) tells us,

"The child's earliest attachments become the prototype for subsequent interpersonal relationships." (p 14).

Certainly when I discussed with Carol her disruptive behaviour in placement her worry was about the placement ending, although Carol's behaviour would then become indifferent to this, saying on occasion that she wouldn't mind moving. It seemed that Carol felt rejected by her mother and the previous placements, and wanted to reject her present carers before she felt they would reject her.

I would have welcomed greater insight into Carol's and her mother's relationship through observing Carol and her mother together, although this was impossible as there was no contact. Similarly, at this point her mother was refusing to meet me, although there was no obvious reason for this. Effectively, Carol's mother had cut her off completely. It seemed that Carol was quite isolated, with a history of lack, loss and poor or negative attachments, with which she was still struggling.

Further indications of attachment issues were demonstrated in Carol's low self-esteem, few outside interests or peer relationships, poor impulse control, lack of trust and low educational achievement (Fahlberg, 1994). In recognition of these difficulties it seemed that much work would need to be done before Carol would be able to move on to a longer-term placement. For Carol to move to a successful future the facilitation of positive attachments seemed essential, as Fahlberg states:

> Once a child has experienced a healthy attachment, it is more likely that, with help, he or she can either extend this attachment to someone else or form additional attachments if necessary. (Fahlberg, 1994, p 18)

Process of the work

Although on most occasions I would advocate a child's presence at meetings, I felt it important to spend some time with Carol's foster carers and with their link worker to discuss how we could assist Carol with her problems; with this aim a meeting was arranged. It felt important to listen to the difficulties the foster carers were having in order to gain insight into Carol's problems, and again to give the input needed to sustain the placement.

The link worker agreed to explore some therapeutic support for the carers themselves; similarly, I felt Carol might benefit from some of her own. I took the notion of the 'positive interaction cycle' (Fahlberg,

1994, p 8) to assist the foster carers in maintaining interactions with a positive focus and discussed what the benefits of these might be in terms of aiding attachment, decreasing behavioural problems and hence assisting the placement.

Carol's strongest relationship was with Ann. Carol demanded a lot and often Ann felt cramped and unable to meet these demands for constant attention. As such we agreed that in addition to trying to increase positive interactions, Ann would create some 'special time' for Carol at regular set intervals to increase this positive reinforcement. This would also assist attachment as a 'claiming' behaviour whereby histories and problems could be shared, helping Carol feel a stronger sense of belonging, although much had been done to incorporate her as part of the family. If Carol was agreeable to the special times they would be reviewed at statutory review meetings. We also discussed the importance of consistency and whether Ann would be able to manage those times.

Carol reacted well to the idea of the special times with Ann, giving her the sense that the two of them had something just for them. It also reinforced that her foster carer wanted to spend time with her, increasing her self-worth and combating what I perceived were negative issues of transference from the mother/daughter relationship. (For a full explanation of the psychological notion of transference see Hjelle and Ziegler, 1985, p 62.)

At the same time I believed that Carol also had other needs. On my visits to her it seemed that she had a great preoccupation with her past and rejection by her mother. Indeed, Carol was confused about much of her past history. Coupled with this was her father's death and her confusion over how to grieve for the father she had loved but who had abused her, and the guilt that she felt for disclosing this abuse. Similarly, Carol had received no therapeutic support over the sexual abuse she had survived. Indeed, the disruptive behaviour Carol displayed may have borne a relationship to her abuse and trauma, as is well documented by many studies (for example, Wyatt and Powell, 1988) in which Peters notes that:

> The demonstrated risk factors for sexual abuse – such as lack of closeness with parents (Finkelhor, 1984) – represent deficiencies ... that may themselves contribute to later psychological difficulty. (p 102)

Given the above, I discussed the potential benefits of counselling support with Carol and we agreed that I should make a referral to the local child and family consultation clinic. In recognition of the perpetrator of sexual abuse being a male, and the issues of transference (see Hjelle and Ziegler, 1985) and powerlessness that counselling may re-engender, a specific recommendation for a female counsellor was made. These issues were also important to recognise throughout my work with Carol. As Carol's sister Jane had also experienced sexual abuse from the father, I asked the counsellor and Jane's social worker if joint sessions could be explored.

Following an assessment meeting with Carol, her foster carers, Jane, her social worker, the female counsellor and myself present, joint counselling sessions were agreed. I felt positive about this as I felt contact with Jane would combat feelings of isolation and blame and also promote what attachment Carol and Jane had to each other. It was agreed that these sessions would be to focus on the losses and bereavement Carol and Jane had experienced, and particularly their past sexual abuse by their father and uncle; a date was set for review. The contact between Carol and Jane acted as a catalyst to increase contact between them, which became regularised to additional monthly contact visits, alternating between where each young woman lived.

Life story work

I felt positive that Carol was now receiving a more focused progressive service, but was still aware of the gap in Carol's understanding of her history and how she had arrived with her present carers. Following a meeting with Carol and others involved in her life we agreed to undertake life story work with Carol. I believed that until Carol had a sense of her past she would have difficulty moving to a new placement, as Ryan and Walker (1985) state:

> A life story book is an attempt to give back to the child in care his or her past life through the gathering and discussion of the facts and people in that life and to help him or her accept it and go forward into the future with this knowledge. (p 5)

Carol was keen to get started and on my next visit had purchased a large photograph album to contain her work. We mapped out the next six visits I would make, with the last one being a review date. Visits were approximately every one-and-a-half weeks to help give a sense of flow and continuity.

Given Carol was developing an increasing attachment to her foster carers, plus their knowledge of her, we agreed that when the work on the book commenced the carers would also be present. I hoped that this would help create a greater attachment and also help the carers to feel included and continue to offer positive reinforcement to Carol.

Preparatory work, although time-consuming, was worthwhile. Initially I again familiarised myself with the case files; a copy of Carol's birth certificate was sought and the hospital contacted for details of birth weight, time of birth and length at birth. After several planned and unplanned visits Carol's mother answered the door, and gave me the few photos she had of Carol's life to copy for her life book. Advantageously it felt that this visit reopened communication with her mother.

As a next step Carol and myself went out to visit and photograph the hospital and previous foster homes; Carol's foster carers also assisted with this work. Visiting these places gave a sense of reality to Carol about her past and, as I have often found, young people talk most candidly in the car! Carol described her feelings about where she had lived, the surprise of what the hospital looked like, and continued to talk about what it must have been like for her as a defenceless baby. At times I would take photographs of Carol outside the various places, at others Carol would use the camera herself.

For myself, it dawned on me how important it was to recognise that different social work methods work for different people. Issues had been raised for me in thinking how another similar young woman with whom I have worked had mostly found it useful to sit and talk whenever we met, and initially I had expected that this might work best for Carol too. Clearly Carol found it difficult to talk sitting face-to-face in a room, but the use of a creative medium really helped.

Further preparation was made in consulting Carol's counsellor to ensure that the life work could go in tandem with the counselling sessions. The added benefit to this was some consultation being offered on how to move through the work. Once we felt all the information possible had been collected we began the regular sessions with the foster carers in starting the book. Boundaries of confidentiality were agreed, and that it was Carol's book and she should keep it. Carol decided that she would wish the book to start at her birth, so that is where we began.

The first pages covered her birth certificate and Carol drew how long she was a baby, as well as sticking in a letter from the hospital. Times of year always held significance for Carol and we talked about how cold it must have been when she was born. As the book moved on so did Carol's memories. Sometimes Carol's memories would not be correct; for instance her memories of her oldest brother whom she had never met. At such times gentle correction was given and dates and events recorded in the life story book, for example through her family tree. As there were few photographs Carol was encouraged to draw events such as the journey to see her eldest sister in a children's home, which she remembered. At the end of this the name and address of the home was inserted.

Certain events, such as the reason for her eldest brother and sister's removal, were difficult to explain, but it was important to be honest. Carol listened intently to recounting of events and would often skip back to earlier parts of the book, should further clarification be needed. To give factual information and further Carol's exploration of her feelings towards her past, a genogram was compiled. Dates of birth and dates of leaving home were added. Significantly Carol's mother's age of leaving home at 15 was added.

This gave the opportunity for us to discuss Carol's mother and some of the difficulties she had. These were not used, however, to excuse her mother's constant rejection of her. I encouraged Carol to express her feelings about her family with felt-tip coloured pens. Carol emphatically stated that the colour red was for those she hated and blue, her favourite colour, was for those that she loved. We discussed what the word 'hate' meant for Carol and she related much about anger and rejection. Carol used red pen for her mother and brother Robert, and for the rest of her family she used blue.

Even though Carol had not truly known her eldest brother and sister she said she loved them. There seemed a sense of allegiance between Carol with these siblings as they too had been abused within her family system. The pictorial representation of love/hate within Carol's family seemed extremely clear cut. I suggested to Carol that I believed love and hate could coexist and invited her to incorporate this in her genogram if she wished.

A small splash of red felt-tip was added by Carol to her father. Carol said that this was due to the sexual abuse she had suffered. It surprised me how forthright Carol was over this. I felt positive that Carol was able to share these feelings and that she was able to externalise and apportion responsibility for the abuse to her father. I interpreted the minimal use of the red pen for her father as signifying hope, although I was less clear still about her feelings towards herself.

Once over the age of five years, Carol's book progressed around the places she had lived and the schools attended. Carol could express some good memories but usually these were tainted by something bad happening later. She recalled the various times she was physically abused by her mother, whereby the foster carers and myself were able to express how difficult that must have been for her and reaffirm adults' responsibilities to care for children. I believed that this had a particularly therapeutic effect.

As the sessions progressed we reached Carol's initial reception into foster care. This proved helpful in explaining Carol's perception of why she was looked after. Carol said that she had left her mother due to arguments before her mother "got rid" of her. It is again interesting to note the pattern of Carol disrupting placements, and that often she would force the end of the placement by her behaviour and then request to leave. This pattern was discussed with Carol, as well as acknowledging the difficulties that Carol and her mother had. Carol's present carers were then able to reinforce their feelings for Carol and how much they cared for her.

Moving on

In the midst of this work a potential long-term placement was located for Carol. After two long meetings with the potential carers I had initial feelings that they would adequately meet Carol's needs. Subsequent meetings between the present and potential carers were set up, with similarly positive feelings. Following completion of the matching report and foster panel approval, Carol was advised of the potential placement. Due to pressure of placements and the need for Carol to start a new school term at the beginning, there were one-and-a-half months left. On my next visit Carol had not completed some tasks on her life book to which she had previously agreed, and said that she would prefer to continue the book in her new placement. This request was respected for, as Ryan and Walker (1985) comment, "If you force the pace, the life story book will become unpleasant for the child and that is not what you want" (p 18).

Carol was now faced with the task of moving. Prior to informing her of the potential placement, an introductory plan had been made as required by departmental policy. It had been intended that Carol would see a video of the new carers when she was told of the placement, but due to equipment failure this was not possible. To relieve anxiety for Carol it was proposed that the new carers come to Carol the day after she was told. As much focus as possible had been placed on Carol's involvement with this plan. Carol wished to change some dates on the plan and these were agreed. Fahlberg (1981b) gives two major means of minimising the trauma of moves:"...giving children permission to have feelings and explaining what is happening to children when they are moved" (p 17).

I spent time with Carol at one–and–a–half week intervals to explore how she was feeling. Carol understood why she had to move and said she liked the new carers, although understandably felt worried by the change and the perceived loss of her present carers, friends she had now made and familiar surroundings, given her new placement was not in the locality. Equally Carol felt guilty for liking the new carers, as she felt this betrayed the attachments she had made.

Introductory visits progressed to overnight stays. Planning was felt to be important, with as long a transition period as possible, given the attachment that had formed. Post placement visits were also planned and agreed, with Carol being aware that her carers had kept in contact with young people they had fostered before her. I believed that pre- and post–placement visits would aid the grieving process and help transfer and sustain the attachments she had made. Carol's carers agreed to come to her new placement also, for us to complete the life story pages which related to her placement with them.

In recognition of Carol's responsiveness to direct work, two further sessions were arranged to assist with moving on. The first related to Fahlberg's (1994) 'three parents', and the second was used for the 'candle ceremony' (p 149).

Within the three parents session we discussed what had been given by Carol's mother and social services, and then focused on Carol's foster carers. A good discussion ensued, with Carol saying what she felt her carers had been able to give to her. It felt liberating that Carol was able to express those feelings, apparently without fear of rejection. Carol's carers then stated what Carol had given them. I clarified that I would remain involved once Carol had moved, and would continue to link in and ensure arrangements were made for her.

Candle ceremony

At the next session Carol, the foster carers and myself sat on the floor with blinds drawn. All had viewed this session with positive but quizzical interest. Initially there had been a jovial atmosphere, with the carers joking about chanting and wearing kaftans for this session. This helped relax the atmosphere. Carol lit a candle to symbolise her birth and continued to light a candle each for her mother, father, sisters and eldest brother, her foster carers and then myself, which surprised me. We discussed the love Carol had for her mother and siblings and how she had transferred this to others.

Carol spoke about what people had given her in life. She acknowledged that her mother had given her life but said that there was no love burning between her and her mother any longer and snuffed her mother's candle out. Next Carol lit candles for her future carers and we discussed how we can love and be loved by more than one person. Carol's carers confirmed again that even when she moved, their candle would still burn for her, and she reciprocated by saying hers would too. Together we acknowledged that it was time for her to have the candles lit for her new carers also. This felt helpful, given Carol's worries about liking her new carers and feeling guilty about this, for, as Galley (1988) indicates, "Older children must have been given psychological permission by their former carers ... to make new attachments" (p 64).

Before the candles had burnt down Carol blew them out and lit them again, naming each one whom she loved, with the exception of her mother. Subsequently we took photos of the candles with each person, and then groups with them. These were a fitting end to lighten the atmosphere after what had been some intense and thoughtful moments. We agreed to repeat the candles ceremony when Carol was with her new carers, which I believed would reinforce for her that the love and care for and of others still remained. Carol was collected by her new carers one-and-a-half-weeks later, as planned.

Evaluation and learning

From comparison of the beginning and end of this piece of work I feel that much was achieved. Initially it had felt that there was a strong possibility of placement breakdown for a young woman in a state of chaos, with little planning and inactive and reactive social services intervention. Little cohesion was seen within the networks geared to support Carol. Given the time, theoretical approaches, available research, experience and commitment of the other agencies, a successful care plan was developed and enacted. I was again reminded of the importance of collaborative working with other agencies, to which I received positive feedback from Carol's carers and counsellor. Similarly, through regular social work visits with clear aims in mind, a trusting relationship was built with Carol, symbolised by her lighting a candle for me.

Inclusion of the young person and involvement in the decision making were important themes to be learnt. The value of the foster carers' role must also be seen. I believe that if Carol's carers had not put such an investment into forming an attachment she could not have moved on or been sustained in foster care. It all seemed significant that with a firm care and visiting plan, crises seemed far fewer and more containable. Referral for therapeutic support had also assisted Carol, with emotional space outside of her placement with a gender specific counsellor, as well as the assistance the carers needed therapeutically to sustain Carol.

Prior to this piece of work I had little experience of direct work with children or young people. Indeed I now feel I had unconsciously avoided it as I had feared it 'wouldn't work' and I wouldn't really know what to do. The benefits of the life story work had really stood out for me. As well as Carol, the foster carers and myself had also enjoyed it. I felt frustrated that we had been unable to complete this work to date due to Carol's move, and worried that as she did not have as full a sense as possible of her history this might hamper her moving on. I shall surely endeavour to complete Carol's life story book and would hope to explore additional techniques with this work, and shall try to match appropriate ones to each individual child at the same time as continuing my learning process.

Endings are always difficult. I felt that Carol had managed this one well. I feel that she had been aided by being helped with her history, and I was served with a reminder of the importance for the social worker to obtain background information. I had always tried to give as much explanation as possible to Carol as to why she would have to move from her short-term placement, which helped. Again, theoretical approaches and wide reading helped me in facilitating a positive ending. Similarly, the 'candle ceremony' about which I was previously sceptical stood out as an excellent symbolic way to facilitate Carol's emotional move. I can see many useful applications of this way of working.

Carol had made great successes in placement emotionally, behaviourally and educationally. I hope that these gains are resilient enough to combat the deficits of the emotional deprivation and physical and sexual abuse she had suffered. To be given every chance of this, Carol did need a long-term placement which would also allow the work that I started to continue, for, as Thoburn reminds us:

... to be able to develop new and satisfying relationships as an adult, the young person needs ... a permanent placement – with the security, sense of belonging ... and loving that go with it – combined with knowledge about his/her family of origin ... and the interconnections between past and present. (in Fahlberg, 1994, p 373)

Sarah:
Understanding and containing damage and disturbance?

Veronique Faure

Position at the outset of the work

Social work with area teams (I work as a senior practitioner in a children and family team in a London borough) offers great potential for varied and interesting work. In child protection work, however, the stress level is such that there is often resistance to working in a creative way. But there is room for it, as my work with Sarah shows.

Sarah (white British, four-and-a-half years) has been on the child protection register for a year under the category of emotional abuse. An initial investigation into possible – but not substantiated – sexual abuse by her father, Jimmy, revealed that Sarah was subjected to an extreme level of verbal/emotional abuse from her mother Kim (see genogram, Figure 1). Enquiries into the family background revealed Kim's very traumatic childhood (with a care history and issues of sexual, physical and emotional abuse), and previous involvement from another local authority in relation to care and adoption proceedings on Kim's other two children.

Kim, from a very young age, has suffered from irritable bowel syndrome to such an extreme that she leaks faeces most of the time. Like Kim, Sarah soils, which triggers Kim's abusive behaviour. Since Sarah's first registration there have been various referrals and investigations, the latest being two months ago when Kim reported hitting Sarah hard and roughly rubbing soiled knickers on her face. Sarah was subsequently placed with her paternal grandparents, where she remains.

Figure 1: Genogram

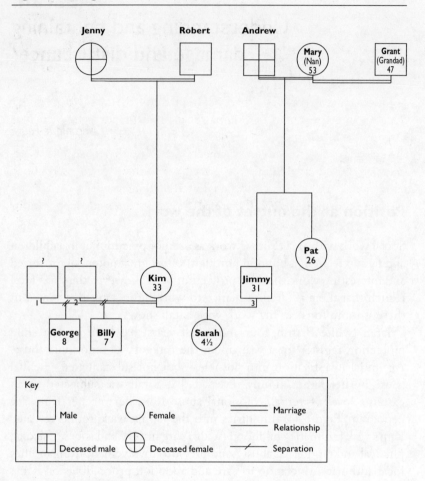

At the outset of the work:

- the case was allocated to a social worker;
- Sarah had been referred to the child psychologist but there was a long waiting list;
- she had been attending nursery full time for three months;
- both parents had been offered counselling at the family centre (not taken up);
- the grandparents had requested to be assessed as foster carers and receive financial support;
- Sarah saw her parents separately at weekends at the grandparents' home.

Three months after Sarah was placed with them it was decided that the Department would not recommend the grandparents as foster carers.

The allocated social worker at the time felt that the family dynamics were such that the grandparents were put in a position were they experienced a loyalty conflict between meeting Sarah's needs or Kim and Jimmy's needs. This caused much distress.

The social worker was also concerned about the fact that in doing her fostering assessment she found out that the grandmother's current partner (Sarah's main carer) had been sexually abused as a child and that the grandmother's previous partner (Jimmy's father) had also been sexually abused as a child. The social worker was concerned about sexual abuse within this family and Sarah's vulnerability.

Due to the above, the grandparents applied for a Residence Order in relation to Sarah and obtained it in July 1996 with the support of both parents.

The social worker had extreme difficulty containing the parents' and grandparents' demands and was unable to offer Sarah any individual input. I was asked to undertake up to eight sessions of direct work with Sarah.

Assessment of the situation: negotiation of the intervention

My assessment is based on a model presented by Dr Glaser during a Goldsmiths course lecture on emotional abuse, which recognises forms and dimensions of ill treatment (Glaser et al, 1994). From what I read in Sarah's file I believed that Sarah was a child who was not recognised (especially by Kim) as an individual who exists in her own right. This was evidenced by:

- Kim's persistent negative attributions to Sarah (describing her as "evil, too powerful, manipulative, dangerous"); her inappropriate expectations from Sarah (generally); her failure to recognise Sarah's individuality; her use of Sarah for the gratification of her own emotional needs.
- Sarah's behaviour at nursery: aggression towards other children, hitting out over toys for no apparent reasons; being bossy; ordering children to carry out instructions; answering for them; sulking; swearing; blocking staff; constant verbal chatter; soiling; lack of concentration. Sarah's soiling (which has no medical explanation), as well as her behaviour, seemed to 'mirror' her mother's, as she shifted from being

a demanding although quite powerless child, to becoming a very controlling and demanding adult. Details of the case suggested an extreme level of projection/identification[1] within the mother/child relationship. The assessment was at a stage where everyone recognised that Sarah could not safely return home.

I have chosen to focus in this case study on trying to understand the child/mother relationship. I will not address the assessment of the father/child or grandparents/child relationships or the issues relating to child protection and possible sexual and physical abuse, but they were constantly present in my mind throughout the work. The work I negotiated with Sarah was about giving her a safe space where she could explore her feelings/emotions through play, and giving myself the opportunity to assess the degree of harm to Sarah caused by her experience of abuse (I felt this was the area that had not been yet assessed).

I agreed with my manager and the allocated social worker that I would only do direct work with Sarah, with no other involvement with the family or in case management. I negotiated regular consultation from the child psychologist (children and family consultation services) on the work that I would do. I had then to think about the venue for the sessions. I did not think that either my office or the family home would be appropriate. I negotiated with the nursery the use of their portacabin, which is independent from the nursery and offers the use of two separate rooms. I agreed to see Sarah on Fridays after the other children left at midday.

I discussed the above with both Sarah's parents and grandparents, who welcomed individual work with Sarah. I asked Sarah's grandparents to explain to Sarah before I started working with her that she was going to see a 'special adult' for a few weeks who would see her at nursery to do some 'special play' and have 'special talks'. I chose to use the term 'special' as I was aiming to give Sarah a different experience of a child/adult relationship from those she was used to at home and at nursery, and to give her the sense of being 'special'.

Theoretical and experiential influences

The Children Act (1989) emphasises the social worker's duty to ascertain and take into consideration children's feelings and wishes before making decisions and planning their current and future care; hence the need for direct work with children. From my own and other practitioners' experience, however, one of the main difficulties is about helping children to verbalise and articulate their feelings and wishes.

Damaged by their experiences of abuse, children often feel confused, disempowered and unable to 'talk' about how they feel and what they want. In current social work practice, one of the alternatives to 'talking' has been the use of 'play therapy' techniques in direct work with children, although social workers (including myself) struggle with the limitations of their competence and training in this area.

Play therapy

The potential benefits of play are well documented in the literature:

> Schaeffer (1980) states that one of the most firmly established principles of psychology is that play is a process of development for a child. Play has been alternatively depicted as a mechanism for developing 'problem solving and competence skills' (White, 1966); a process that allows children to 'mentally digest' experiences and situations (Piaget, 1969); 'an emotional laboratory' in which the child learns to cope with his/her environment (Erikson, 1963); a way that the child talks with 'toys as his words' (Ginott, 1961); and a way to deal with behaviours and concerns through 'playing it out' (Erikson, 1963). (Gil, 1991, p 27)

The theory and practice of 'psychoanalytic play therapy' was first formulated in the 1930s by Anna Freud as "a way of building a strong positive relationship between child and therapist", and by Melanie Klein as a "direct substitute for verbalisation" (Gil, 1991, p 29). In my work with Sarah this is how I intended to use play: to engage her and build up a trustful, safe and strong relationship between us; as a way of helping her express what she could not verbalise, as well as helping myself gain some insight into her internal world and conflicts.

From what I know of Sarah and Kim's relationship and of the powerful game of projection/identification leading Sarah to be/act like a 'little Kim', my reading of *The drama of being a child* (Miller, 1993) had a tremendous impact on my insight into this mother/child relationship:

> There was a mother who at the core was emotionally insecure, and who depended for her narcissistic equilibrium on the child behaving or acting in a particular way. This child had an amazing ability to perceive and respond instinctively, that is unconsciously, to this need

> of the mother [for the child] to take on the role that had unconsciously
> been assigned to [her]. This role secured 'love' for the child.... [She]
> could sense that [she] was needed and this [she] felt guaranteed [her]
> a measure of existential security. (Miller, 1993, pp 22-3)

Miller further writes about children who have developed "the art of not experiencing feelings, for a child can only experience feelings when there is somebody there who accepts him fully, understands and supports him" (p 25). This I felt could be one of my roles in my work with Sarah, giving her an experience of an adult who could accept her without judgement or pressure, respect her, not make emotional demands on her or expect her to behave in a certain way for the gratification of the adult's own needs.

I thought that to achieve this I would try to work in a way that I had not really experienced before, that is, in using non-directive play therapy techniques (as opposed to directive). From my reading of relationship therapists such as Virginia Axline (1947), I decided to be as non-directive as possible, allowing and encouraging Sarah to choose what toys to play with, and giving her the freedom to develop or terminate any particular activity.

Dibs: In search of self (Axline, 1964) had a very significant impact on my choice of work. I was powerfully attracted by the simplicity of Axline's non-directive stance in relation to Dibs – how deceptive, however, as my evaluation of my work with Sarah will demonstrate. I can smile now at my naïvety, but my reading of *Dibs* did not prepare me for the powerful feelings that Sarah stirred up in me, although containing those feelings is central to non-directive play therapy.

Anti-discriminatory framework

My local authority has a strong commitment to equal opportunities and anti- discriminatory/anti-oppressive practice. This is very much reflected in the child protection procedures which are "written within a feminist anti-discriminatory framework" and "recognise the difference in power held by men and women", do not see parents as "an amorphous group, but as individual women and men", "seek to enhance the status of women, who form the majority of carers of children" and "treat mothers in sexual abuse work as our allies in protecting and caring for their child" (Local Authority Child Protection Guidelines, 1992).

This, in Sarah's case, is particularly worth noting as she first came to our attention following an allegation of sexual abuse. Somehow in the process of the investigation this was partly lost and the workers focused on the emotional abuse Sarah was subjected to by her mother, partly because it was displayed in such an obvious and extreme way.

Society, and sometimes children and workers themselves often blame mothers of sexually abused children for failing to protect their children, and they are almost portrayed as responsible for letting it happen. In Sarah's case, Kim might have not only failed to protect her child but perpetrated abuse herself in quite a shocking way. The child protection conference reflected the workers' concerns about this "awful" mother and placed Sarah on the register for emotional abuse, failing to address the other facets of a very complex case involving issues of possible sexual and physical abuse. Similarly, I question my choice of focus in this case study on the emotional abuse aspect.

The allocated social worker for Sarah was black. In our discussions throughout the work, we acknowledged the impact of dealing with fairly powerful, and sometimes abusive, white service users, as well as my position of authority as a white senior practitioner in our co-working relationship. I must also note my own anxiety in any work I undertake about being a foreigner, and children struggle sometimes with my French accent, although I never felt that this was an issue in my work with Sarah.

Process of the work

I had one introductory and seven further sessions of work with Sarah, and arranged two more sessions to end the work. I had three consultation sessions with the child psychologist and arranged a professional meeting attended by Sarah's grandparents. I have had no contact with Sarah's parents, but had a few brief conversations with her grandparents, as well as with the nursery key worker.

I have had regular supervision from my course coordinator, one session with my team manager, and regular discussions with the social worker to ensure sharing of information, consistency of work and of messages given to the family, and sharing of feelings and difficulties encountered in the process of our separate work.

My sessions with Sarah were never easy and were charged with powerful emotional content both for her and for myself. Some sessions were very enjoyable for both of us and some very frustrating, sometimes leaving me with strong feelings of helplessness which I identified as a process of counter transference[2] of Sarah's feelings.

Evaluation of the intervention

During my first introductory visit to Sarah there was an almost immediate rapport. I had asked her grandparents to prepare Sarah for meeting me. She was expecting me and engaged straightaway in talking and drawing. This first contact was easy, and highlighted the benefit of good preparation and planning with all involved. Sarah always welcomed me with a big smile on all my further visits and was clearly pleased to see me. I will only elaborate at length on two main areas drawn from my evaluation of the intervention, and mention some of the other relevant areas.

Play/activities within the sessions

Paint and clay

During my first session of work Sarah chose to do painting. The nursery worker had brought us some paint but the only colours left were red, brown and black. I feared that these colours could be associated by Sarah with her soiling. However, she wished to carry on painting.

From behaving well at first and using the brush, Sarah transformed (after I allowed her to finger paint) within seconds into a fairly wild and extremely controlling little girl, pouring paints on the paper and smearing them with her hands, demanding to paint my face (which I refused). She got out of hand very quickly, flicking paint on the walls, on the carpets and on myself. We engaged in a battle of wills as I needed to assert boundaries to ensure her safety (physical and emotional) and mine.

At the second session I thought that if Sarah needed to act out issues around her soiling, I could let her express this more safely through playing with clay, which is less messy and said to be a good tool for getting in touch with primitive feelings/emotions (Aldgate and Simmonds, 1988). Sarah played with clay for a few minutes but quickly got out of hand and started throwing clay everywhere and at me. I had to be firm and removed the clay.

With hindsight, and insight gained from my consultation with the child psychologist, I realise that these two situations must have been experienced by Sarah as real 'set ups'. Here I was, trying to provide Sarah with a safe space to explore her feelings, and I had put her straightaway in a very risky, anxiety provoking situation. The paint colours (which I had no control over) were clearly associated by Sarah with faeces. She wanted to smear my face with them as her mother had smeared hers with soiled knickers, as if she wanted to abuse me as she had been, making me as bad as her mother, as powerless and of no use or help to her.

I had assumed that the nursery would have lots of colour paints available and did not check before the session. This lack of preparation/control, the child psychologist felt, was equally, if not more, meaningful to the child than the actual paint colours. I wasn't in control: how could Sarah feel safe? And how much more of a set up was clay? Clay that looks like, feels like, and dries on the skin like faeces. Even if paint and clay could have been used with Sarah to help her act out issues around her soiling, this could only have been done much later on, after feelings of trust and safety had been built up through previous sessions.

The mouse and the bear

During the second session, as I was clearing the clay, Sarah ran off to the other room and closed the door behind her. I worried about what she might be doing/feeling, so I knocked on the door and entered. Sarah was hiding under a small table. I pretended not to see her and 'looked' for her everywhere.

Subsequently a game developed that carried on through most sessions. As I searched for her, she would make a squeaky noise like a mouse, or a roaring noise like a bear. If she was the mouse I'd look for her to keep her safe from the bear. If she was the bear she'd pretend to catch the mouse before me and eat it. She'd swap from one to the other, depending whether she needed to be the helpless, scared vulnerable little mouse (the child), or the powerful, frightening controlling bear (the adult, the mother).

Her facial expression and body language would change dramatically and I could see the fear or the rage/anger on her face. She would repeat this game endlessly across sessions. I was initially surprised by Sarah's interest in this repetitive game, usually more age appropriate for toddlers, especially as Sarah is a very bright and articulate child, able to get involved in very elaborate activities. This game, however, seemed to have different functions for Sarah.

First it allowed her initially to test out whether I cared enough about her to look for her and ensure she was alright. Also it gave her the opportunity to play as a younger child, with no demands or expectations that she would have to achieve. The child psychologist pointed out that Sarah's articulateness and brightness were likely to be defence mechanisms that Sarah had developed to protect herself. Maybe she felt safe enough with me not to need them.

The bear eating the mouse rather than just killing it is worth noting, because of the association between eating and defecating/soiling. By eating the mouse Sarah was also able to rid herself of some of her fear and vulnerability. To give Sarah the mouse to look after at the end of our sessions until the following week was, I believe, very meaningful and positive. It acknowledged to her my understanding that she could be both frightened and frightening. It also reinforced the message that I wanted the mouse, the vulnerable part of her, to be safe and protected.

In the fifth session Sarah was able to feel powerful enough to kill the bear again and again, getting rid of the aggressor. I thought this was a positive move. The child psychologist, however, pointed out that although she was killing the frightening, controlling bear, she was also identifying with an even more powerful aggressor – the hunter needing prey. Sarah already had a tendency to control and bully other children at times.

The issue of soiling/wetting

Sarah soiled or wetted during most of our sessions, I believe as a result of addressing powerful feelings or difficult situations. The nursery workers and grandparents had done a lot of work in encouraging Sarah not to soil. The grandparents especially felt at one time that they had to demonstrate that they could care for Sarah better than her parents, and one of the signs was that Sarah was almost not soiling anymore. Instead Sarah suffered from constipation for weeks for which she had to receive medical treatment.

The issue of soiling/wetting was the most difficult and sensitive to deal with. Sarah's experience of soiling since she was an infant had been dealt with very inappropriately by her mother especially, because of Kim's own issues and traumas. She acknowledged never having been able to clean Sarah without feelings of disgust and anger, even when Sarah was a baby.

I felt it was important in my session to deal with issues of soiling or wetting with as much normality as possible and not make a 'big deal' out of it. I felt very strongly that Sarah's soiling had gone beyond the possibility of attention seeking and had become something that she actually had no control over, and was a response to overwhelming emotions triggered by stressful situations. I felt that soiling needed to be dealt with not as 'good' or 'bad' behaviour but just as a normal bodily function.

The patterns I identified were at times when I had to be firm with her and ascertain boundaries (going to the portacabin or going back to the playground), when she felt invaded (her grandparents walking into the room unexpectedly, her hand being held very tight) or when we had to end sessions. Sarah's initial reaction when she wetted or soiled herself was one of either anger projected at me (hitting me), or shame (hesitating to tell me). This to me was a sign that Sarah had some positive sense of self-esteem and pride and cared about herself.

Sarah initially would not ask me to clean her, and declined my help. The turning point was in the fourth session when Sarah soiled after I had forced her back to the playground. She was angry, hitting me and shouting "Leave me alone". When we got to the toilet she told me to stay outside. After a while I offered to help her; she declined saying she could do it herself but then asked me whether I could make sure her bottom was clean, and let me clean her properly.

I felt that Sarah was initially angry with herself for soiling, wanting to 'fix it' herself, with no help, trying to take the responsibility for her soiling. I understand Sarah's soiling as maybe a way (unconsciously) of making herself 'smelly', messy, to make people go away, reject her, or punish/abuse her. However, I didn't leave her in her soiling, did not run away, get angry, threaten her, hurt her or blame her. By staying around and offering my help again, I gave her the message that I cared and might be able to help, that I was able to contain and hold her anger and that I could survive.

By asking me to make sure her bottom was clean she moved from wanting to fix it herself to acknowledging that maybe she could fix it better with me. I therefore was not just a part of her. At the next session, when I got to the nursery, Sarah told the other children "That's Veronique" – a real, separate person from her.

During my last session with Sarah, when she soiled and I told her that it was "no big deal", she replied that her granddad was going to tell me off for saying that. This full acceptance of Sarah, including her soiling, raised some difficulties with her grandparents about giving out different messages. I arranged a meeting with the child psychologist, the grandparents and the other professionals involved to discuss the issue, as the psychologist believed Sarah was not confused about the messages she received and knew they had different meanings for different purposes.

Ground rules and boundaries

In initiating work with Sarah I told her I would be meeting her to play in "whatever way she wanted". When Sarah and I engaged in a battle of willpower during our first session she told me in anger "You said I could do what I wanted!": a fair interpretation of what I had said. By the end of the session I had made new ground rules and told Sarah that for our work to continue we must agree on safety with each other. Therefore, I would not allow her to hit me or hurt me or throw things at me or elsewhere, and that I would equally not hit her or hurt her.

I asked Sarah to repeat the rules several times and asked her grandfather to remind her of the rules during the week. Issues of safety and security are always important for children who have been abused and I realised that my own feelings and sense of security and safety (which I did not always have) were equally important if Sarah was to feel safe.

Sarah carried on testing boundaries. During our fourth session, for instance, she ran out of the playground into the street. We ended up in another battle of wills as I had to be physically quite forceful with her, which made Sarah extremely angry. I was aware that this could remind her of past abusive situations and make her feel emotionally very unsafe, although it had to be balanced against her physical, therefore emotional, safety.

Significance of the venue of the sessions

In planning the work with Sarah I thought the nursery would be safer (because independent) than home or the social services office. It was a shock when I was told at the last session that the portacabin had been previously used for interviewing Sarah during an investigation of child protection issues! How unsafe it must have felt for her. With hindsight it helped me understand why Sarah was at times extremely unsettled, trying to avoid going to the portacabin or being reluctant to answer questions.

On one occasion Sarah insisted on playing outside and I allowed this to happen. The child psychologist pointed out the importance of always keeping to the same venue to ensure consistency and boundaries, and therefore emotional and physical safety. He questioned why I had not insisted on going into the portacabin. I realised that I had been worried about getting into another battle of wills with Sarah. He pointed out that Sarah probably wanted to avoid getting into the room to do some work and deal with powerful and uncomfortable feelings, and that I had colluded with the avoidance for probably the same reasons. It was more fun to play outside, less threatening for both of us.

Another difficulty Sarah and I encountered was about keeping the venue safe by ensuring privacy and preventing others from interfering and invading the space. One good example of this was during our sixth session, when Sarah's grandparents walked into the room 20 minutes too early to pick her up, which provoked Sarah's anger.

Ending of the work

I have arranged for two more sessions of work with Sarah, who does not attend nursery anymore and has started school in her grandparents' area in a different borough. I will visit Sarah at home after school and will negotiate with the grandparents some privacy and respect for Sarah's time and space with me.

In my work with Sarah very powerful feelings were aroused, both for her and for myself. Because of their strength I believe the relationship between Sarah and me became a strong one fairly quickly, although I have only met with her on eight occasions. I am conscious of my own feelings of sadness at the prospect of saying goodbye to Sarah, as part of me wishes I could deepen the work further.

I am also aware that Sarah might not facilitate the process of ending, and might feel/be angry with me or even reluctant to acknowledge that it is the end. It will be important for me not to collude with Sarah's likely avoidance and to share my own feelings. I have booked a further consultation with the child psychologist to prepare for this.

Learning from the work

Consultation with the child psychologist and supervision from my course coordinator have been of extreme value and allowed me to address with a degree of honesty (and without blame) the failures and successes of the work undertaken. They facilitated this by offering me a safe space and valuing my work, while making constructive criticism that helped me move from a fairly 'frozen' position at times.

I realise that my wish to provide a therapeutic input within this setting was a bit ambitious, given the limited nature of my contact with Sarah and her history. The main aspect of learning here is about acknowledging the difference between my strong wish to rescue Sarah/make it better, and the constraints one works under.

The quality of contact between Sarah and me, however (notwithstanding the frustrations), was, I believe, good throughout and I learnt that this more than anything enabled the situational shortcomings to be managed: I clearly enjoyed Sarah in her own right, and I believe Sarah appreciated this and responded.

I learnt from the guidance I received to identify issues of transference and counter-transference. I see the main transference at the start of the work, when I felt at times mostly a part of, a reflection of Sarah, that Sarah found quite hard to give up. This developed when I had to stand for a potentially punitive or even perverse maternal figure, although there was an acceptance of a more kindly maternal figure with whom Sarah could be messy (and be cleaned), without shame.

As for the counter-transference, I felt at times quite powerless and angry with myself (especially when I failed to ensure emotional safety or keeping of boundaries). My anger and powerlessness could be in part a projection of Sarah's, having spent much of her life always being in the wrong and fearing to mess things up. I learnt (the hard way) how to survive as a 'therapeutic presence'. This was threatened by being unable to guarantee the security of the therapeutic set up, and by being (psychologically and physically) attacked by Sarah. For example, the episode of painting my arm shows how the 'messing' can make somebody one's own (no separateness). My 'survival' as an independent person becomes evident in latter sessions when Sarah acknowledged me as a separate person and let me clean her.

I have learnt that attending to a child's confusion and distress is different from reacting to it, and learnt to 'stay' with Sarah's pain and anger without always lapsing into wanting to be 'reassuring'. I learnt from the reassurance I received from the child psychologist that as long as one responds to a child with genuine respect and honesty, social workers cannot damage children in their direct work anymore than they have been already.

I have learnt a great deal from Sarah herself in allowing her to lead me in her play, in establishing a trusting relationship with her and in being aware of her growing attachment to me. As a result of this piece of work I feel I have now more resources, both internally and externally, to understand and work with children's experiences and deal with their pain. I have confirmed my conviction that direct work techniques are important and worthwhile as an aid to social workers, and I have been able to transfer some of my overall knowledge and understanding into practice. As my realisation of this and my experience increased, I have felt more effective and confident as a practitioner.

I learnt that doing direct work with children needs careful preparation, planning and organisation, and benefits from the use of others' skills through consultation and supervision. I feel I now need to deepen those areas of learning, through theory and practice, and learn how to share my learning with other practitioners, especially those I supervise.

I also plan to start attending the children and family consultation service peer group discussion around direct work.

Notes

[1] *Projection*: "In the properly psycho-analytic sense: operation whereby qualities, feelings, wishes or even 'objects', which the subject refuses to recognise or rejects in himself, are expelled from the self and located in another person or thing. Projection so understood is defence of a very primitive origin."

Identification: "Psychological process whereby a subject assimilates an aspect, property or attribute of the other and is transformed, wholly or partially, after the model the other provides. It is by means of a series of identifications that the personality is constituted and specified."

[2] *Counter transference*: "The whole of the analysist's unconscious reactions to the individual analysis and especially to the analysist's own transference."

Transference: "For psycho-analysis, a process of actualisation of unconscious wishes. Transference uses specific objects and operates in the framework of a specific relationship established with these objects. Its context par excellence is the analytic situation. In the transference, infantile prototypes re-emerge and are experienced with a strong sense of immediacy."

Commentary from an academic perspective

Kate Wilson

Therapeutic intervention, in the sense of providing sensitive helping professional relationships, continues to be at the heart of good social work practice, despite the somewhat case-managerial approach to practice which seems to have developed over the last decade. I have been interested in therapeutic social work practice since beginning my career as a probation officer, and worked with adults with marital difficulties at a time when it was still an accepted part of the probation officer's role to do so. Much more recently I have focused on child therapies, exploring ways of undertaking what has come to be known as 'direct' work within a statutory context.

Following a short period as social worker and team manager in a local social services agency, which made me aware of the need for post-qualifying training in childcare, I set up a post-qualifying programme in child protection at the University of Hull. As part of this, we introduced a component of non-directive play therapy, and began to develop ways of using this approach in statutory settings. The approach itself is based on Rogerian client-centred therapy with adults, adapted to working with children, and uses play rather than verbal exchange as the principal means of communication.

I moved to a new post in the social work department at the University of York, where, together with my colleague Virginia Ryan, who has the main teaching and supervisory role on the programme, I set up a two-year, part-time MA/Diploma in non-directive play therapy. When we started the programme, we were uncertain as to how successful it would be in the current climate. It is now in its sixth year, and the fact that it continues to recruit well-qualified and committed social workers (along with others from different professions) seems some evidence of the continuing interest among social workers in therapeutic work with children. I also teach on the University's Master in Social Work course, and am currently involved in a research project on supporting foster placements, funded by the Department of Health, which is looking, among other things, at the provision of therapeutic services to children and young people in foster care.

Although I have a specialist interest in non-directive play therapy, I am keen to encourage the continued involvement of practitioners in a variety of direct work with children and families: historically, much therapeutic work has been undertaken by social workers (and indeed major therapeutic innovations have derived from social work practice), and it seems worrying that the role of the British social worker in local authority social services departments is becoming more that of a case manager and less of a direct worker. This may lead to a distancing between worker and clients, and the loss of casework skills which should be the hallmark of the good practitioner. On our social work qualifying programme at York, we try to make the development of these practice skills central to the social work training, and it is therefore good to see, in these accounts of work undertaken as part of the Goldsmith's Advanced Social Work programme, practitioners using a range of approaches to direct work with children and young people.

Although meeting with varying degrees of success, all show a willingness to become engaged with the emotional life of the children/ young people they are working with, and to be open to trying to understand their particular worlds. They convey well some of the complexities of childcare practice and the way in which the best laid plans can become derailed. There are some pointers to good practice which emerge from the accounts. Some of these are familiar and may seem obvious, but one of the advantages of these 'real life' accounts is that they show how it is possible to omit stages which – with hindsight – may seem perhaps obvious in preparing for and working with the children and young people.

The cases all show how essential it is to make an overall assessment of the child's problems and situation, before deciding to work directly with the child. This assessment may identify a range of needs which should be addressed, by different kinds of therapeutic intervention, as in the three-pronged approach described by Stephen Kitchman. It may also indicate that advocacy rather than individual work is more urgently needed, as in the case described by Patrick Lonergan. The assessment must include the quality of the relationships between young person/ child and carers: first, essentially, to ascertain that the child is safe; then that his/her attachment needs are at least minimally met: and thirdly, if individual work is to be offered, to ensure that the carers will be supportive during therapy, and can be guided in how to do this appropriately. The assessment also needs to take into account timing in relation to the ongoing plans for the child; the amount of time required to complete the work and the worker's skill and experience, in relation to the level of difficulties shown by the child; and the therapeutic goals of the intervention.

Once the decision has been made to undertake therapeutic work, it is important to ensure that this individual work is integrated into the child's or young person's overall environment, rather than being kept separate from the family system, as seemed to be the case in some of these accounts. It seems to be harder to do this when the practitioner has to combine the roles of therapist and case manager, and Michael O'Dempsey's account illustrates this difficulty, which will be familiar to many trying to do direct work in a non-specialist setting. Equally, practitioners need to be clear about the different roles of the professionals involved, and recognise that it is essential to coordinate their work in helping the child and family.

Finally, as Patrick Lonergan's case study shows especially, the practitioner's relationship with the child or young person is necessarily a personalised one. Non-directive play therapy in particular, but to a lesser extent the other approaches to direct work described here, are based on a highly empathic attitude and a deliberate intensifying of adult–child interactions. It is very easy, particularly when things are not going well for the child elsewhere, for practitioners to overpersonalise the already close relationship, perhaps entertaining 'rescue' fantasies or overstepping their professional role in other ways, and it is essential to be able to address these issues through good supervision.

Patrick Lonergan
James: Moving on to independent living

As the writer himself candidly acknowledges, this is a flawed, and in the light of the goals he set himself when undertaking it, largely unsuccessful intervention. However, for all its inadequacies, it does bring to life some of the complex processes involved in working with the emotional relationships between the young person, their carers and the wider environment. The language frequently used to describe social work and childcare practice in particular can be misleading, giving an over concrete picture of 'packages' of care, and suggesting an objectivity, a rationality and detachment which disguises the personal, emotional dimension which the practitioner inevitably brings to the interaction. In this case, the worker only belatedly recognises that at least some of the difficulties he has had in supporting James' transition into independent living have occurred because they reflect current personal difficulties over endings.

Even leaving aside this transference, he refers to feeling 'an enormous responsibility' and 'almost like a father figure' as he contemplates transferring the case, and his intervention highlights many of the emotions which are often consequent on highly personalised adult/child helping relationships – a feeling of responsibility and powerlessness, a fear of getting things wrong, and a desire to make things better or to rescue James from the troubling situation he has been placed in. It is useful to be reminded that childcare practice is a dynamic process: it helps us in part to understand how mistakes are made, information missed which in retrospect seems obvious; and challenges the ultimately unhelpful view that practice can be fitted tidily into a specified framework.

This said, it does seem that the approach to working with James before he leaves care was misconceived. The practitioner is – with reason – critical of his agency's policies in relation to young people leaving care. James is established and settled in his current foster placement, and having to move on at this juncture is arbitrary and not, on the information given, in his interests. (See research findings, reviewed, for example, in Stein, 1997, which conclude that placement stability, continuity and some family contact are strongly associated with successful outcomes for young people leaving care.)

Young people leaving care have a statutory right to after-care until they are 21 and under Section 24 of the Children Act (1989) there is permissive legislation for resources to be made available which might have enabled him to remain longer in his foster home. Biehal et al (1995), however, report a wide and regrettable variation in the way in which different local authorities interpret this legislation. In other words, a full assessment of James' needs should first have been made, followed, if indicated, by an attempt to secure alternative support. One feels that by the time this possibility is raised at the review meeting, the inevitability of a move has been tacitly accepted by those involved, despite their sense that this is designed to meet agency requirements rather than James' needs.

The underlying principle of the direct work with James is, I think, that in order to move on successfully to the next life stage, past experiences need to be understood and integrated in the personality. Using the attachment framework referred to in the early part of the case study, this intervention seems inappropriate: even though he has apparently overcome early attachment disruptions, and seems to have developed a secure attachment to his current carers, this 'secure base' is now under threat, making it unlikely that James would feel emotionally free enough to undertake the challenging explorations which the worker plans and which, in any case for anyone, seems likely to be painful without some careful mediation.

In the event, both parties quickly recognise that this is too difficult for James at this stage, and the plan is abandoned (reminding us that it is often easier for adolescents to exercise choice than it is for younger children). The contact in the remaining weeks is disorganised, yet one feels that the final meeting did achieve something of the good 'ending' which the worker had originally intended, and the account ends, justifiably, on a note of optimism.

Mary Cody
Eve: From victim to healthy survivor?

This account usefully illustrates the fact that the provision of a stable and loving new family may be insufficient to enable a child to overcome the effects of earlier multiple abuse and deprivation. As the writer concludes, there has been a tendency to view the provision of post-adoption services as cost neutral, and there is anecdotal evidence that adoptive parents still may have difficulty in accessing help when they need it, months or even years after the adoption.

A study by Thoburn (1990) suggests that intervention in the early period after the adoption when the child and family are still settling in may not be appropriate, but that, as here, in the longer term, therapeutic help may become necessary. Difficulties, again as here, classically arise or become less containable, in early adolescence. We are not informed about the aegis of Eve's problems, or the quality of the family relationships, a point I shall return to. Nonetheless, the problems are highly stressful for young person and family alike, and ready access to effective support for them becomes a moral imperative.

Having acknowledged the appropriateness and timing of an outside intervention, what of the intervention itself? The writer seems to be attempting what we have described elsewhere as a 'therapeutic assessment' (Ryan and Wilson, 1996, ch 7, 2000a: forthcoming, 2000b: forthcoming) that is, a time-limited intervention in which the practitioner develops a therapeutic relationship with the child or young person, and through this relationship reaches a clearer understanding of the child's developmental needs, wishes and feelings. Potentially, such sessions are of immediate benefit as they allow the young person to explore important personal themes to therapeutic effect. In the longer term, they clarify her/his future needs, including therapeutic ones, so that an appropriate range of support can be devised. The purpose of the work is described initially as one of empowerment, and later as achieving an understanding of Eve's feelings, although the writer seems unaware of this shift. The framework suggested above would have been helpful, partly in ensuring that the assessment component is adequately realised.

We are not given much detail of the structure and content of the sessions, but may infer that a range of structured techniques and exercises were used. In the case of the narrative story stems described here, they seem to have been effective in engaging Eve, and may well have been helpful to her, as well as providing some clarification of her self-concept and hypotheses about her likely defences against emotionally difficult experiences. Since it is indicative of Eve's developmental stage, which needs to be part of the assessment, it is worth noting that the story stems referred to are designed for a younger age group. It is, of course, important to use age-appropriate techniques, especially with adolescents, who can quickly become bored or disengaged. The limitations of such techniques, in addition, are that they can be used inappropriately (risking, for example, breaking the child's defences), and that because the adult determines the focus, the concerns which the child addresses are those identified by the adult rather than the child.

It is disappointing that having with some success developed an understanding of Eve's inner world, the assessment is so loosely tied in with future plans. A fuller assessment initially of the family might have ensured better integration, and also the vital involvement of the adoptive parents in the progress of the intervention. For example, the first session poignantly supports the hypothesis that Eve has attachment difficulties, here displaying a pattern of anxious attachment to her adoptive mother. These attachment issues need to be addressed with them both, particularly in helping Eve's mother to understand and meet them in a way which addresses Eve's anxieties and her mother's own needs. (see Downes, 1992, where she explores interactions in adolescent foster placements within an attachment framework, is particularly helpful here.) Ideally, this work would go in tandem with individual, time-limited therapeutic sessions for Eve, conducted by a different practitioner.

Michael O'Dempsey
Amos and Christopher: Working towards care proceedings

This intervention divides into two parts: the first eight sessions are designed as therapeutic assessments (see my comment on Cody's case study); the purpose of the remaining six sessions, although unstated, is, one assumes – broadly therapeutic – to help the children and their mother manage their feelings as they re-establish their family relationships and adjust to their father's lessening involvement.

The intervention, particularly in the first stage, seems to have been helpful for both children. The practitioner clearly got to know and understand their world, and the children trusted him and were able to communicate their feelings about themselves and their wishes about their future clearly. He responds sensitively and appropriately to them: for example, when Amos expresses sadness at having no one to help him, he reflects this feeling and goes to find him when, overwhelmed by this, Amos leaves the room. He is critical of his subsequent response to Amos, which he considers overly rescuing. Although perhaps true, it highlights the dilemma of combining the two roles of therapist and key worker: the former needing to help Amos clarify and master his feelings, the latter needing additionally to consider future plans.

Clarity about his role as therapist might have enabled him to stay focused on Amos' feelings: for example, 'You do want people to help you, but you're not sure that can happen', rather than becoming, as he apparently was, preoccupied with concerns for Amos' future. The difficulty of combining the two roles is particularly evident when the possibility of a child protection investigation arises, but is a contributing factor in some of the problems which occur after the children's return to their mother. Although a common problem in conducting therapeutic work in a social services agency, it is worthwhile separating the two roles, if at all possible.

Greater attention needs to be paid, in both components of the intervention, to the quality of support from the children's carers. It must be established that they provide an at least minimally acceptable environment, and are able to support the child in working through emotional experiences which may emerge during therapy. When undertaking an assessment of children in foster care, whose experiences will necessarily have involved some degree of disruption or loss of permanent parenting figures, the practitioner needs to be cautious in attributing all of the child's emotional problems to past trauma, and must be alert to the possibility that the difficulties are due to current care. (See also my comments on Faure's case study.)

On their return home, it would have been helpful to clarify the purpose of continuing therapeutic sessions with the children's mother, and to establish a pattern of support for and from her during the sessions. In structuring a play therapy intervention, it is the practice on our play therapy programme at the University of York to ask that the carer brings the child to the play room and waits during the session in an adjacent room. (For a discussion and illustration of setting up and conduction play therapy sessions see, for example, Wilson et al, 1992; West, 1996; Ryan and Wilson, 1996). This reassurance that their carer is nearby is important for all children embarking on the anxiety-provoking experience of therapy, and provides an additional security if, as may occur particularly in early sessions, the child wishes to leave before the full hour is up.

In attachment terms, their carer's presence provides a secure base from which they can embark on emotional exploration. Given Amos' and Christopher's experience of disrupted attachments, and likely anxieties on return home, it would be essential to secure their mother's ongoing commitment, and without this to rethink the appropriateness of the venue and even the value of the sessions themselves at this critical juncture. Filial therapy, such as that described by Guerney (1984) or Van Fleet (1994), or some family sessions with mother and children at home, might have been alternative approaches.

Stephen Kitchman
Carol: Moving to a permanent placement

This account focuses on some direct work which followed an assessment of a 13-year-old girl in foster care. Carol's needs were hypothesised to include problems with attachment and a need to develop a more secure attachment with her main foster carer and, possibly less crucially, with her sister; her need to resolve feelings over the sexual abuse she had experienced; and the need to identify past experiences so that these could be understood and the emotions involved addressed.

The account illustrates well the way in which a successful intervention must be preceded by a full assessment and may form only part of the required response. In attachment terms, the plan for the foster carer to enhance Carol's feelings of security by establishing some regular special time between them seems highly appropriate, and in turn this increased sense of security is likely to have enabled Carol to engage in the counselling and in the life story work. This three-stranded approach surely helped Carol to make the successful transition to her new foster carers.

The choice of life story work seems appropriate to the chief task of adolescence, namely the reintegration of past experiences into the current sense of self and the gradual development of an adult identity. For Carol, as for many adopted and fostered children, this process is made more difficult because they have to rely on their own partial and incomplete memories, as well as having to come to terms with the premature separation from birth families, and the inadequacy of these adults as role models. The timing and approach of this work, at this age and while she is relatively settled in her current placement, is therefore well-judged.

The practitioner is sensitive to Carol's wish to put the life story book to one side as she prepares to move into a new placement, and recognises that her more immediate needs are to explore her mixed feelings of anticipation, guilt and apprehension as she does so. The symbolic means chosen of lighting candles seems perfectly judged for a 13-year-old girl, and again indicates that the adults concerned were tuned to her world, gender and needs.

In his evaluation, the worker suggests that this period of Carol's time in care was characterised by careful planning and a coordinated response. This included cooperation between the different agencies, a purposive and regular pattern of social work visits and support, the appropriate involvement of Carol's carers, and the well-judged use of counselling and activity-related therapeutic approaches such as life story work and metaphors. I would add that throughout, the approaches were characteried by a responsiveness to Carol's feelings and a recognition of what would be appropriate to her situation and to her developmental age, and that this allowed the development of an enabling therapeutic relationship.

The evaluation concludes that this planned work was probably vital in helping her to become sufficiently stabilised in her current placement to be able to move on to a permanent one, a conclusion with which I wholeheartedly agree. The time and resources required must at the time have seemed considerable, but are negligible in comparison with what would have been required had the placement broken down, as must at one time have seemed likely.

Veronique Faure
Sarah: Understanding and containing damage and disturbance?

This account of eight play therapy sessions conducted with a disturbed four-and-a-half year old raises a number of concerns about the appropriateness of undertaking the intervention and the methods used. The practitioner describes her approach as being "as non-directive as possible", but it would be unfortunate if this was seen as an illustration of non-directive play therapy.

Before undertaking play therapy, it is vital to form an assessment of the child's overall situation, to establish whether or not the carers can provide a minimally secure and responsive enviornment for the child. At the very least, one needs to ensure that the child's attachment needs are being met, since without this stability, it is unlikely that she can entrust herself to therapy, and indeed may look to the therapist to meet these needs. In Sarah's case, however, in the light of information about their history, one would be concerned about her grandparents' ability to protect her from further abuse; indeed, Sarah's current male carer has himself two high risk factors as a perpetrator, and one would expect him to be the subject of a separate risk assessment before Sarah was placed in his care. It is disturbing that having been turned down as relative foster carers for Sarah (which does not extend to general approval), the grandparents then successfully obtain a residence order for her.

Thus the first concern should be Sarah's safety with her current carers, followed, only if this is satisfactorily established, by an assessment of their ability to understand and respond to the emotional impact of the therapeutic work on Sarah herself. We have, in the example of Sarah's game of mouse and bear, an illustration of the importance of assessing her current situation as well as informing oneself of her past history. Any hypothesis about the meaning of a child's symbolic play can by its nature only be inconclusive: however, here we have no way of judging whether Sarah's play is more likely to reflect, say, her mother's earlier abusive behaviour or possible aggressive responses from her current carers.

In addition, it is also important to have an introductory meeting with the carers, not only to engage their support for the child during the intervention and alert them to possible difficulties (for example, a child may become messier or more badly behaved during therapy), but also to gain basic information from them about the child. Here, there were issues around the management of Sarah's toileting which needed to be clarified to try and avoid the difficulties which did indeed arise from differing approaches.

A third issue to be addressed concerns the practitioner's level of experience and training, and whether or not these are sufficiently developed for the particular demands of the case. On our play therapy training programme at the University of York, we would only expect students on their third placement to work with a child showing Sarah's level of disturbance. We find that a common wish on the part of beginning students and their seconding agencies is to work with the more damaged and needy children. Although understandable, this is a mistake: practitioners need to have developed sufficient skill and understanding of the approach before they can work successfully with the kind of problems such as limit testing shown here.

To her credit, the worker became aware that her preparation for the intervention was inadequate. Axline's books (1947, 1964), although providing a delightful and vivid introduction to non-directive play therapy, do not address current issues arising from statutory work or consider the family system or other contextual issues, and are insufficiently detailed about practical considerations of setting, preparing the playroom, transport and so on. The early difficulty about the failure to provide appropriate materials is a reflection of this lack of information. (See Wilson et al, 1992; West, 1996; and Ryan and Wilson, 1996 for a fuller discussion of case management and practice issues.)

As she acknowledges, the worker is also ill-prepared to meet the difficulties of setting limits with a child whose behaviour quickly becomes out of control when the framework of the sessions is not clearly set out and consistently maintained. She recognised her mistake in suggesting that there will be total permissiveness – indeed Sarah astutely identifies this herself. If a child is to engage on emotionally troubling issues, it is essential that she feels safe and contained. Good practice usually involves explaining limits of permitted behaviour (not hurting self, therapist, breaking toys etc), limits to confidentiality, and some rules, for example, to do with time limits for the session and leaving the play room. (See Landreth, 1991 for a useful discussion of limit setting and the therapeutic as well as practical implications.) Carol's account of her work with Kelly, age six, who had recently moved to her current foster placement, also provides a helpful account of a short non-directive play therapy intervention following an assessment with a child in the care system (1998, pp 85-90).

Commentary from a practitioner perspective

Rosemary Gordon

Introduction

Before providing a commentary from a practitioner perspective, it may be helpful briefly to describe my own background and approach to direct work with children. I shall also describe how I approached the task of providing a commentary on these five case studies.

My professional background is in probation, where latterly I worked as a divorce court welfare officer during the early 1980s. This experience had a profound impact on me, coming at a time when a fresh approach to family conflict resolution found a voice in conciliation. Work in a team that adopted the principles of conciliation, and applied them to situations of family conflict within a systemic framework, began to achieve startling results that avoided the damaging impact of Court-based decisions. The approach began to recognise the value of children's contributions – if used carefully and sensitively and avoiding the court-induced imperative of 'Who would you rather live with?' We began to involve children more and more in the decision-making process, developing communication skills through training and practice.

This experience demonstrated the necessity of helping children make sense of their circumstances past and present, express their feelings and wishes, and contribute to any decision-making process. These principles I carried into child protection work in the NSPCC, as a team manager and then trainer of practitioners and supervisors.

In summary, my approach to working with children combines the application of the major theories of childcare, the value of a systemic framework, and a constant questioning of assumptions based on discrimination and the mis-use of power. My current interests lie in exploring our conceptions of childhood and how these are played out in the systems and structures we employ for them, working inclusively with children, and achieving a balance of rights for children linked with a sense of responsibility – for their families, schools and communities.

A recent role has been responsibility for the development and production of training and resource packs. I was first involved with the consortium that produced *ABCD: Abuse and children who are disabled* (NSPCC et al, 1994), which resulted in a greater inclusion of disabled children. Working with a small group who developed and produced *Turning points: A resource pack for communicating with children* (NSPCC, 1997) was an opportunity to bring together much of the knowledge, skills and understanding relating to working with children and young people. Some of the references in this commentary have drawn on its comprehensiveness and accessibility, although it should be recognised that further reading in particular areas is essential.

Currently I am involved with the development and production of the Department of Health's training pack *The child's world: Assessing children in need* (NSPCC/University of Sheffield, 2000), supporting the Framework for the Assessment of Children in Need and their Families. This provides practitioners and their managers in all the relevant agencies with a systematic approach to assessment that builds on research, theory and good practice.

Approaching the task as a commentator, I began by reading each case study carefully, absorbing the content and being aware of its impact. Next, I read it again, making notes as I began to apply knowledge of theory and practice, and of practitioners, to the studies. I then returned to them later, re-reading them thoroughly and drawing together the themes already identified and placing these in what I hope will be a helpful framework for the reader. The task was absorbing and owed much to the ability of the authors to convey their affection for and understanding of the young people with whom they worked so carefully.

Patrick Lonergan
James: Moving on to independent living

Patrick accurately identified the two main themes facing James – separation and loss, and transitions – without recognising that they currently mirrored his own life. This is only too easy. His early preparation was good: he discussed the piece of work with James and negotiated extra time with his manager. Despite identifying the two key themes – both inviting exploration of feelings – the work was initially planned in a task-centred way, by looking at past files. It could be supposed that this was unconscious avoidance of feelings, but in any case the exercise had enormous impact on both James and Patrick. It evoked many painful memories for James, and for Patrick the recollection of his attachment for James, as well as the recognition of the similarity to his own personal life.

The application of attachment theory was appropriate, although Fahlberg's (1994) work may have been of more value in its application to placement endings. Equally I would have been interested to know how James had been helped to overcome his early poor experiences of parenting and to understand his particular coping strengths (see Gilligan in *The child's world*, NSPCC, University of Sheffield, 2000). This may have helped in the planning process of moving on. I would guess that Patrick's long and committed involvement had much to do with it, and some exploration of this might have helped Patrick to identify his worth to James.

Patrick's reading around separation and loss was good and he had clearly given much thought to the likely processes (see Jewett, 1984). What he had not been able to envisage was the impact of visiting these painful areas of James' past. Patrick showed respect for James by not wishing to push him further. This is a frequent dilemma for workers – how to balance the desire to empower the young person and help them gain control over their lives, with the knowledge that there are unresolved areas that 'need' further work. Patrick's task-focused solution is understandable, although he was again avoiding the emotional issues. Avoidance and drift was inevitable and the work was in danger of collapsing. By stirring up so many feelings it is possible that James felt that his past was so bad that Patrick would change his opinion of him and not want to see him again.

There is also the sense of the work being driven by outside forces – the procedure and systems for leaving care. This also had the result of further avoidance of the real issues, and leaves one questioning strongly the timing of leaving care services (see Fletcher in *Turning points*, NSPCC, 1997). Young people are faced with huge choices at a time of experiencing feelings of fear of the unknown, being unprepared and often very lonely. To change a known and trusted worker at such a time is questionable in the extreme. Equally, to expect the worker to shed the sense of responsibility that has shaped the value of the work is also unrealistic.

Patrick's description of how the work revealed identical processes for him in his personal life is painful to read, and his determination to face his own loss and stay with James through this time is admirable. However, he desperately needed good support and supervision, and it is not clear from the account that this was adequately skilled or forthcoming

(Hawkins and Shohet, 1989; Brown and Bourne 1996). It is possible, with hindsight, that co-working might have helped. There is a sense that Patrick was left on his own to identify the processes and needed permission to acknowledge the validity of his feelings and be allowed to grieve properly. Additionally, it might have helped James to have his mother more closely involved in the work and thus able to share some of the painful memories with him, as well as to include the new worker more actively, thus giving James permission to form a new attachment.

Patrick showed insight into the question of gender possibly being a feature of their previous task-focused relationship, yet the relationship clearly provided James with important boundaries and structure. The actual 'ending' ceremony went well, although I came away wishing there had been a 'transitional object' to acknowledge the transition part of the loss process. Patrick has been of enormous importance to James and a tangible reminder of this might have comforted him.

Mary Cody
Eve: From victim to healthy survivor?

In this piece of work it would have been easy to collude with Eve's perception of being 'the problem' and to confirm her self-perception. In the face of a potential adoption breakdown, it would have been easy to respond reactively to Eve's destructive behaviour and lack of impulse-control.

Fortunately Mary avoided this, and instead adopted a child-centred perspective on Eve's history and present difficulties. She established a conceptual framework, starting with a review of attachment theory (Fahlberg, 1994; Howe, 1995) and the development of defence mechanisms, connecting this to Eve's likely feelings and past experiences, and linking it to her developmental stages.

Mary is in touch with her own feelings about the work from the outset, and alert to the likely psychological processes that would occur in her relationship with Eve, such as transference. She is able to bring her inexperience of this to supervision. Working on one's own emotional issues is a vital part of preparation for this work and the ongoing nature of it. Past emotional losses or pain need to be acknowledged, preferably through good supervision, since they often only emerge when provoked ʼır children or situations (Hawkins and Shohet, 1989; Brown e, 1996). Workers need to be as clear as possible about their ional boundaries, both to protect the child and to protect themselves from inappropriate feelings and responses. Mary demonstrated an ability to reflect on this objectively, while legitimising her intuitions about Eve's feelings. Her plan to 'create space to listen' to Eve is an excellent approach.

Having begun to hypothesise about Eve's unmet needs and likely feelings, Mary then reviewed the case records. I liked the analogy of the empty emotional 'bank account'. Again, she anticipated that this process would be painful and used supervision appropriately. In the course of the review Mary noted Eve's resilience and her coping mechanisms (see Smith in *Turning points*, NSPCC, 1997 and Gilligan in *The child's world*, NSPCC, University of Sheffield, 2000). This gave valuable clues as to future work with her. Mary had explored the family's perspective on the current difficulties and harnessed their understanding and support. Similarly, she facilitated Eve's empowerment by allowing her to plot the sessions and negotiate a 'contract'.

By gaining understanding of the power of transference and projected feelings, Mary is able to experience the full extent of Eve's despair. The recounting of particular incidents, as well as the careful use of story stems, showed Eve's cognitive distortions of her experiences and a central negative belief about herself. Her inability to hear praise, let alone to believe good things about herself, showed a schema of defectiveness, being unlovable and incompetent (see Lavender in *Turning points* and Young, 1990).

As the work progressed, Mary is able to recognise many of Eve's childhood experiences as traumatic. Her observation that "these memories are laid down in a part of Eve that has no words" is correct. Young children who are traumatised develop extraordinary memories. If they don't understand something they move closer to look. If they have no explanation or interpretation, without words the image remains fixed. The emotional memory of the pre–verbal child has no words for the troubled adolescent and is therefore prey to the sudden replaying of early trauma.

Mary demonstrated her empathy and understanding of Eve's distress in her response to the row Eve had with her mother. To respond to her like a small child and then to use relaxation and breathing techniques is a good example of intuitive practice. She recognised the playing out of traumatic memory and was able to hold and contain it both for Eve and for her mother, using it as an opportunity to affirm their feelings for one another.

This is an excellent piece of work, in my view, using the three routes to understanding, as described by Mary. The material is vivid and painful and yet the worker, by careful assessment, planning and use of supervision, has offered Eve a safe and structured opportunity to explore her past and make sense of her present. This is in line with the new Assessment Framework. Clues to future work may lie in greater exploration of resilience and Eve's coping strategies by the application of cognitive behaviour therapy at some later stage. This is a hopeful model in that it conveys the message that change is possible by offering an alternative perspective. The work ahead is difficult and lengthy: Mary is correct in reminding us that work such as this cannot be hurried.

Michael O'Dempsey
Amos and Christopher: Working towards care proceedings

The presenting problem in this family was the separation and divorce but, as with most severely acrimonious separations, this merely provided a different route by which existing deeply experienced problems were played out. Michael was quick to identify the other issues, all of which had already had an impact on the children. This was a family with a high octane level of functioning; domestic violence was regularly witnessed, as was verbal and racial abuse of the mother by the father; emotional and physical abuse of the children (see NSPCC et al, 1998). The mother's own mental health problems had resulted in earlier separations and losses for the children, before this, the latest one. Both boys also showed responses common in children who are frequently 'carers' by showing huge loyalty to and protection of their mother. Cleaver et al's (1999) recent review of research into the impact of parental problems such as domestic violence, mental illness and drug and alcohol misuse would have been of value here in assessing the impact on the boys' developmental needs.

It would have been easy to focus on the divorce and the issues of residence and contact, to the exclusion of past issues. Michael's background reading on attachment, domestic violence, Erikson's model of the development of identity, and children's experiences of divorce and separation helped him to understand the children's presenting behaviour and place it in a context (see Dasgupta in *Turning points*, NSPCC, 1997; Wallerstein and Kelly, 1980; Wallerstein and Blakeslee, 1989). During periods of intense confusion and anxiety, children's behaviour, no matter how bizarre, mostly makes sense when viewed through their eyes. They are usually trying to piece together the bits they can control, or attempting to exert some control or mastery over the bits they feel responsible for, that feel out of control.

Thus one of the first challenges was to set realistic goals within an appropriate theoretical framework, and place practical and emotional boundaries around it – both for the children and the worker. Michael sought support and understanding of the work with the foster carer as well as with the mother. This was important since the work would inevitably raise issues for the boys that would emerge after the sessions. Another strength of Michael's approach is to recognise and avoid the temptation of finding solutions for them. In this situation, the needs were so entrenched and so complex, the initial goals needed to be modest.

Michael was careful in his choice of methods and techniques, using background reading to understand play as communication and to distinguish different approaches. He is right to be initially concerned about Amos' potential splitting of his personality in the first session, and to identify this as indicative of his intense difficulty in coping. It is likely that this was a traumagenic state caused by reaction to the witnessing of violence towards his mother, and was possibly an early indication of a dissociative disorder (see Kaplan in *Turning points*, NSPCC, 1997). This is common in attachment-impaired children who face traumatic episodes such as this.

A further significant theme that emerged was the complex construction of a family belief system around racial identity (see Banks in *Turning points*, NSPCC, 1997). The denigration of the mother's racial identity (against the existing social background of racism) was overlaid with the attributing of the boys' physical racial characteristics to either the 'good' or 'bad' parent. Michael's acceptance of their identity and the work on positive reinforcement showed promising results through Amos' use of the multi-racial dolls.

The other key theme that runs through all the sessions is the boys' experience of loss and separation. Both boys showed different stages of loss and Christopher, in particular, was 'stuck' at the stage of yearning and pining for the family he fantasised about, and the family he had lost (Jewett, 1984).

In summary, the key elements to intervention in this complex situation were a knowledge and application of attachment theory, recognition of identity confusion, and of post-trauma stress reaction. The support that Michael sought and obtained for himself through supervision and consultation is vital in a case such as this. The impact on him of the boys' reactions and the interplaying of processes needed skilled and sensitive interpretation. Michael's insight into his own occasional difficulties is illuminating to himself and to the reader.

Stephen Kitchman
Carol: Moving to a permanent placement

The initial reaction to this case study is how hard it must have been for Stephen to identify a message of hope for Carol – let alone himself. The situation had all the ingredients of placement breakdown, as Stephen accurately identified from research and guidance, coupled with a history of no planning, assessment or care plan. The situation was chaotic, mirrored by the chaotic state of the files. It would have been easy to continue this reactive process by hastening the next placement.

It was essential to stop, take stock of the situation and attempt to bring some order into Carol's world. Stephen demonstrates that he was able, in supervision, to voice his concerns about Carol, and draw on back-up knowledge about relevant research in order to obtain necessary space. He again used research from child abuse inquiries (DoH, 1991a) to support his intention to spend time on collating an accurate chronology of her life. This review revealed the serious attachment deficiencies that marked Carol's early years and provided the clue to appropriate intervention. His approach to assessing her needs is in line with the new Assessment Framework (DoH, 2000).

Stephen used attachment theory in his analysis of Carol's past and present difficulties, locating them accurately in the rejecting relationship with her mother and then in the abusive relationship with her father. He used Fahlberg's (1994) checklists to assess Carol and planned his intervention on the premise that once a child has formed a healthy attachment she may be able to extend this to someone else. This gave him (and Carol) the much needed message of hope.

Stephen is careful to place the work in a context of partnership and empowerment, with Carol's present foster carers and link worker. He redressed the previous poor networking by involvement of the link worker. Using Carol's present strongest relationship, with her foster mother, he suggested they spend some 'special time' together to try to increase some positive reinforcement. It would also address the poor previous mother/daughter relationship Carol had experienced, and hopefully be a building block for future attachments.

Once Stephen began his work with Carol he identified further issues that needed attention. Again, it would have been easy to react and attempt to deal with everything. He recognised her confusion and ambivalence towards the father who had sexually abused her and the outstanding treatment issues (Sgroi, 1982). Somehow she would need to allow both the love and hate towards her father to co-exist. I particularly liked Stephen's decision to involve her sister in this work and the care with which he negotiated a sensitive gender match in the selection of a counsellor. In involving her sister, he removed a potential source of 'victim blaming' and promoted further positive attachment possibilities.

The main focus for Stephen is undertaking life story work and again he demonstrates the value of careful planning. He recognised that in moving on, Carol would need to understand her past. He involved her carers, recognising the importance of their views about how parents should behave. He allowed Carol control over the process, again addressing her low self-esteem. Stephen showed how a worker new to some of the techniques can, with careful preparation, provide an effective and sensitive communication.

In summary, this careful piece of work has shown how a situation in which a young woman in danger of yet another placement breakdown, due to inactive and reactive practice, can be retrieved. The new Assessment Framework (DoH, 2000) would be of value here in reassessing a situation that had probably been subjected to many earlier assessments. A care plan that separated the attachment needs from the therapeutic needs achieved the necessary space for Carol and the worker to prepare her adequately for the transition to her long-term placement. Although it isn't made explicit, I hope that Stephen had adequate supervision, given the impact on him of this sensitive and painful piece of work.

Veronique Faure
Sarah: Understanding and containing damage and disturbance?

This piece of work was well prepared, despite awareness of the resistance to undertaking creative work in a busy child protection team. Sufficient space was negotiated to undertake the work and, most importantly, consultation with a child psychologist. It is to the author's credit that she persisted in both her background reading and her personal supervision throughout the course of the work, which became increasingly complex and demanding.

Veronique began by extracting evidence from the file about the mother's perception of Sarah and of Sarah's behaviour. Both gave serious cause for concern. There is a sensible focus in the planning in identifying the modest goals of creating a safe space for Sarah to express herself; and assessing the degree of harm caused to her. In fact only one of these goals was realised, although the material would significantly contribute to a full assessment later. Again, the new Assessment Framework (DoH, 2000) would have provided a more systematic and thorough means of assessment of all Sarah's needs.

Veronique's exploration of 'play' as a method of communication is thorough. She acknowledges her lack of confidence in this area but recognised that the particular presenting problem, of Sarah's mirroring of her mother's soiling, suggested that a non-directive approach would be best, using Miller (1993) and Axline (1947) for guidance. This was wise; in the face of such entrenched behaviour, a more directive approach would probably be the preferred option of many workers, hoping to modify her behaviour. Veronique put this issue to one side (although she ran into difficulties later over negotiations with the grandparents), intending to provide Sarah with an example of an accepting adult. This she did, although again running into problems, this time with boundaries and ground rules. All these issues were taken on board and brought to supervision for guidance; an excellent example of the value of ongoing consultation and support (Brown and Bourne, 1996).

I think perhaps reading around attachment disorder could have alerted Veronique to Sarah's inadequate or non-attached attachment needs (Howe, 1995). This could have been used more explicitly in providing Sarah with an example of a positive attachment, from which she could move on with greater confidence. However, the theoretical influences drawn from psychotherapy were appropriate and the interpretations were used carefully. Veronique was alert to issues of transference and clearly gained a deeper understanding of these processses.

The preparation for the direct work is thoughtful and careful, borne out by the ready engagement of Sarah (see Bannister in *Turning points*, NSPCC, 1997). However, Sarah's reaction to what was later interpreted as a 'set-up', and her subsequent regression, was unexpected and could easily have thrown the worker off course. Added to this was the emotional impact of the work on Veronique, for which she was unprepared. This little girl was constantly testing out, and soiling had become the vehicle through which control was exercised (by Sarah, by her grandparents, by previous workers). Veronique is right to choose a different route to establishing trust, consistency and reliability. The issue of the previous use of the portacabin could not easily have been predicted, yet it seemed like something else to thwart the progress of the work.

One of the main learning points for Veronique seems to be in the resistance to 'rescuing'. Resolving conflict between the pressure to be emotionally available and the need to retain objectivity and provide clear personal and professional boundaries is difficult, but one in which I believe the worker succeeded. The work was successful in terms of providing a therapeutic input for Sarah – probably the first she had experienced. Veronique did provide an emotional space in which to tolerate this child's powerful feelings and this was crucial in terms of her beginning to feel understood. With careful attention to the ending of the work, Sarah should go on to apply the positive attachment she made to Veronique.

Conclusion

Reading and evaluating these narratives has been an illuminating and privileged task. The work is of an exceptional standard, thoughtful and sensitive to the children and young people and always mindful of their carers and the wider context. In summarising my own comments several themes repeatedly emerged during each case study and demonstrate, I believe, a foundation to excellent practice. These are presented in the following section as learning points.

Learning points

Rosemary Gordon

- The importance of a sound understanding of attachment theory and its application to all work with children.
- The relevance of an understanding of post-traumatic stress reaction and the likelihood of this being a feature in the history of an abused child. If the right questions are not asked, this can remain hidden.
- The impact of direct work with children on the worker and the absolute necessity of good supervision and consultation.
- The likely interplay of the work with aspects of one's own life.
- A knowledge of the likely psychological processes that may occur, and the opportunity for illuminating this through good supervision.
- The possibilities of undertaking this work in any setting, given the right support and resources, even if there is only limited equipment.
- The value of the primary resources of time, consistency and supervision.
- The value of knowing the research and using it appropriately – whether in arguing for space to do the work or for resources for the work itself.
- The necessity of careful assessment, planning and setting realistic aims.
- The value of working in partnership with parents and other carers.
- The ability to recognise children's resilience and their desire to heal and be healed.

Part 2:
Work with families

Introduction

What is a family? If the answer is not straightforward, why was the requirement to work with a family part of the practice component of the Goldsmiths course?

The nuclear two–parent family living with their dependent children (not too many of them) is now no longer the norm, in spite of what certain politicians would have us believe: for example, one in five families with dependent children is now headed by a lone parent. In the examples of practice which follow we have illustrations of a range of family structures.

For the purposes of the course, the working definition of 'a family' was 'two or more related people of different generations living in the same household'. Even this is a rough and inadequate definition, in that 'the family' can be a powerful reality even when its members are dispersed. As Sigurd Reimers comments, "it is often of greater value to focus on the quality of relationships rather than household composition". So why work with a family? The response must be that the early dependency relationships, in whatever family structure, exercise an abiding influence on the way we live our lives and the families we go on to create. As Mary Cody writes, "the family is the major source of support and stress".

The centrality of systems theory

Part 1 on direct work with children and young people stresses the centrality of attachment theory; in this chapter systems theory, and its relationship to attachment theory, is fundamental, as is a sharp awareness of structured power relationships. These can accrue to almost any aspect of difference and are perhaps most frequently seen in the way gender power is exercised in families. At some level this is a feature of all the work which follows, but most particularly in Michael Atkinson's work with the Reid family.

Both commentators stress that 'thinking systems' is not only appropriate but essential if intervention is to be relevant and effective. In the practice examples we see each author attempting to 'think systems' and apply that thinking in practice while grappling with a range of complex, and often dysfunctional, situations in which children may well be in need and/or at risk. Mary Cody's work, in assessing a family applying to adopt, reminds us of the value of applying a clear theoretical formulation in work which, while primarily about assessment, is also about preparation for a fundamental change in that family's system.

Systems thinking does not just apply to the users of social work services and members of their kinship network; it applies with equal force to the so-called helping network, that is, the agencies and professionals involved, and beyond that to the social environment which impacts on both users and helpers alike. This is a feature of all the work which follows. Sigurd Reimers comments that "systemic thinking encourages us to examine our professional systems (not forgetting ourselves) as carefully as those of the families we encounter". Schuff and Asen (1996) further comment that:

> Conflicting opinions and actions by the various professionals often affect the child and family and cause further disturbance. The family and professionals in turn are very much affected by the social welfare system and fluctuations in child care policy (pp 136-7).

The person within the network of systems can be represented diagramatically by a series of concentric circles (see Figure 1).

Family work teaching

Frequent reference is made in the examples that follow to the course teaching on family work. This comprised only three days in an over-packed curriculum, yet, like pebbles thrown into a pond, the ripples of this powerful teaching (richly illustrated by live material on video) spread outwards to other parts of the programme, and most importantly, through supervision and tutorial work, to practice itself.

The teaching was deliberately entitled 'Work with families' rather than family therapy. There are a number of family therapy courses available; some course members came with this training, others may choose to progress on to it later. The Goldsmiths teaching enabled and encouraged course members to apply systems thinking to the practice of their employing agencies. No one particular approach with its accompanying methodology could be taught at any degree of depth, although various approaches and styles were illustrated on video and

Figure 1: The person within the network of systems

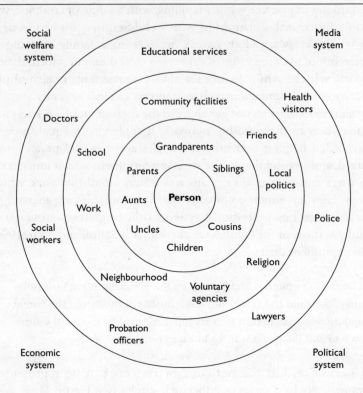

Source: Schuff and Asen (1996)

evaluated in discussion. There is evidence in the practice examples of attempts to apply this teaching, sometimes tentatively, always thoughtfully. It is more difficult to establish how successfully.

Some earlier writings on family therapy (for example, Minuchin, 1974; Palazzoli et al, 1978; Minuchin and Fishman, 1980, 1981; Burnham, 1986) encouraged a certain methodological orthodoxy. Course members, however, were encouraged to apply a range of methods, considered appropriate to agency function and consistent with the limits of the worker's skill and style of work: Patrick Lonergan comments specifically on this. So it is that we see the use of conventional methods such as genograms, ecomaps (Mary Cody, Michael Atkinson), as well as methods such as direct observation (Patrick Lonergan) drawn from other areas of work.

When working across the generations there are considerable advantages in involving family members in a common task and producing something concrete. The course teaching encouraged exploration of new and different ways of working: an example of this is the creative and sensitive use of the genogram. This could be described as the most basic tool of family work but it is also potentially explosive, since family secrets may be exposed and loss and grief laid bare. Children can sometimes lead the way here: six-year-old Joanne Phillips, for example, suggested that the babies who had died in utero (her mother had four miscarriages since Joanne's birth) should be included in their family tree.

The effectiveness of any technique is reliant on the skill of the worker using it; in Mary Cody's work with the Phillips family we see how such material was used and how relevant it was, as the family contemplated adding a new member through adoption. Although the work presented here provides no illustration, a clear visual portrayal, either on paper or through some kind of enactment, can be an appropriate and non-discriminatory way of working with people with a learning or other disability. Talking is not necessarily always the best means of communication.

Effectiveness and outcome in relation to the agency context

The agency's function can operate as a helpful boundary and focus, but can also serve to diversify and confuse the role of the worker. This is apparent in Michael Atkinson's work where the worker had a previous relationship with the family, and in Veronique Faure's where the child protection concerns of the agency had to take precedence. There is a sense in which work in statutory settings may appear more compromised than in clinical settings, limited – as it often is – by lack of resources and a degree of resistance from management. There are also be legal and other requirements which are predominant responsibilities.

Certain questions arise from this: for example, how desirable or indeed possible is it for the worker to assume a neutral position when they are acting as an agent of the state? Furthermore, as both commentators remind us, while positive outcomes are actively sought, they are also elusive. What may be experienced as positive for one or more family members may seem controlling and unacceptable to others; yet social workers must consistently work to ensure that the welfare of the child is the paramount consideration (Children Act (1989) Section 1.1).

Sigurd Reimers refers to social workers working with families as more like explorers than experts. Despite the emphasis on user-led services and working in partnership to facilitate the empowerment of service users, endorsed, for example, in the White Paper *Modernising social services* (DoH, 1998a), many local authorities are still uncomfortable with this approach, believing that they employ social workers to solve problems and to do so as economically and speedily as possible. The futility of this is discussed fully in Smale et al (2000), where an alternative model of practice is presented. This describes how social workers and their managers can tackle problems experienced at the local level by working collaboratively with service users, carers, the wider social network and practitioners in other organisations, to effect sustainable solutions and longer-term social change.

There is an implicit argument here as to process and outcome: if the process of exploring difficulties facilitates the empowerment of the family to address its own problems, this is clearly more effective than where the social worker assumes an expert role which is more prescriptive and potentially disempowering. This approach may well also be rejected by the family. 'Solutions' are sustainable if they are owned by the family and not imposed from outside. Mary Cody writes of the enactment of family dynamics and processes, and states of the Phillips family that "they were able to make connections and develop insights themselves, rather than me taking on the role of interpreter of the emerging data".

This is not to deny that there is a proper and necessary place for the use of professional authority: social work also includes a social control dimension and the worker has certain statutory powers and legal obligations. But the contemporary values of partnership and empowerment sit more comfortably with the notion of the social worker as explorer rather than expert. As Jane Dutton states, "social workers are more often involved in complex processes than in neat final solutions".

In the longer term, the three great 'Es' of the 1990s (Economy, Efficiency, Effectiveness) are more likely to be achieved through informed and skilled exploration. The process may require more resources in the short term, but working to achieve lasting change and independence merit a higher 'E' rating. There is nothing more costly than prolonged and chronic dependence: costly in terms of human suffering as well as resources.

The worker in the agency context

Jane Dutton observes that a focus for each piece of work is the relationship around the presenting difficulty. Agencies are set up to provide service in response to such difficulty, yet problem definition is not a straightforward matter: the definition can often shift when the presenting 'problem' is exposed to the searching gaze of sharp systems thinking. In commenting on Patrick Lonergan's work, Sigurd Reimers underlines the dilemma clients often face, as to "whether to face the discomfort of working at change within their family relationships or to seek a solution (sometimes a distraction) through the use of services". He adds that "in practice either solution may be valid". However, this could only be true if it could be demonstrated that both alternatives would be equally effective.

Stephen Kitchman describes the dirt and disorder of the Dray family's situation and writes "in view of the long history of social services involvement with and knowledge of the family, a continuing response of giving financial support seemed inadequate. Despite case recording of the parents' low abilities, they had become one of the best financed families in the area". How often, and at what level, had the agency ever reflected on the effectiveness of this seemingly reactive, repeated and even routine financial provision? Working in partnership to empower all eight members of the family, as Stephen Kitchman sets out to do, certainly destabilised the family. But this approach also broke through the chronic 'stuck' position, and thus opened up some possibility of change.

All statutory agencies know families with some of the characteristics of the Drays, and who have one or both parents with a care history. Here the social services department becomes like a parent, and risks becoming part of the problem system rather than problem solution. Informed reflection, thinking 'systems', seeking feedback and locating sufficient space to stand outside the system, are all components of effective practice. And if the agencies involved seem swamped by the chaos, it is essential to explore the impact of this on the children who have to live in it.

Both commentators refer to the value of co-work. This was actively sought by at least one of the writers but was not considered possible. In many social services departments it is difficult enough to allocate one worker to acute cases, and the reluctance to allocate two is understandable, though misguided. Working to achieve lasting change may seem unrealistic when the agency is under extreme pressure and functioning in a largely defensive mode in order to survive. Workers, like users, can lose hope and cease to believe in the possibility of change. This issue is addressed by both commentators in relation to specific pieces of work and in their general comments, and discussed fully in Smale et al (2000).

The need for boundaries and supervision

In this context, the worker needs to establish a boundary between the personal and the professional to be able to stand outside the situation: to adopt what Smale et al (2000) refer to as a 'marginal' position, and focus effectively on the needs of the service users. We all have, or have had, families. So it is that situations of lack, loss, dislocated relationships, even abuse, are as likely to characterise the life history of helpers as well as the people they seek to help, although the resources to address these may vary widely.

The role of supervision is critical here and was exercised and experienced in varied ways in the five practice examples which follow, four of which took place in different inner London social services departments and one in a specialist voluntary agency. All formed part of the assessed course work.

Case studies

The Phillips family: an adoption assessment

Mary Cody

Position at the outset of the work

Alan and Melissa Phillips (ages 34 and 33) have made an application to adopt to the voluntary children's agency specialising in adoption for which I work. This is being processed within the relevant legislative and procedural frameworks (1976 Adoption Act , 1983 Adoption Agency Regulation, circular LAC(84)3, agency procedural guidelines). Statutory references have been taken up and there are no contra-indicators to proceeding. Two personal references have also been obtained and are supportive.

The applicants attended two full day preparation workshops for prospective adopters. They are a married white couple with two birth children, Conor (age 9) and Joanne (age 6). I was asked to undertake a home study with the family and to present their application to the agency's adoption panel (see genogram, Figure 1).

Negotiation of the work

The concepts of partnership and empowerment underpin and inform this work. Empowerment of Alan, Melissa and the children began at my first contact and would develop over time. The best way of progressing this is, I believe, to make the work as open and as transparent as possible. Part of this negotiation was orienting the family to how I saw us working together. By being open, clear and honest with them I saw myself as modelling the relationship I hoped we would develop during the course of the work.

Together we looked at our mutual expectations and sought to clarify them. We had a reasonable consensus at this point regarding the time frame and the frequency of our contact. We agreed to meet on a fortnightly basis and envisaged that the home study would take approximately six months to complete.

Figure 1: Genogram

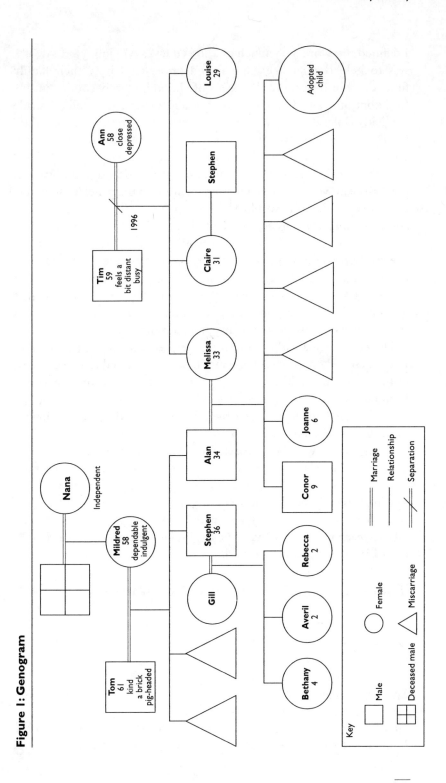

I defined the work very much as a shared task. My job – as I saw it – was to help them make explicit and understand how their family functioned in relation to the needs of children who become available for adoption. I had certain expertise and experience which I made explicit, while also emphasising that they were the experts on their family. I was endeavouring to get them alongside me as curious, enthusiastic co-researchers in a joint venture.

Within this context it was important to acknowledge the issue of power: the power to make a recommendation to the panel lay with me, and to surrender this would be incompatible with safeguarding the adoptive child's best interests. I felt we succeeded in having an open debate around the use of power. I would do my utmost to make the exercise of power transparent by sharing my observations, my hypotheses, my developing thinking and ultimately my report with them. I encouraged a proactive engaged response from them. Within this context we also looked at how concerns and grievances could be addressed and the use of the agency's complaints procedures.

The two essential tasks of the work were assessment and preparation. I saw these tasks as proceeding hand in hand. I wanted to make it clear to the family that neither I nor the agency had some 'normative' family in mind whom we would be measuring them against. Rather, on the basis of a shared understanding of their family and the demands of adoptive parenting, we would come to an agreement about the way forward.

At this stage it was also important to acknowledge the feeling content of the process. Alan and Melissa were able to articulate a whole gamut of feelings from excited anticipation through to uncertainty and anxiety. During this early stage I felt we did reach a common understanding of the process, through identifying shared goals and the steps we would take to reach them. Here were the beginnings of trust and congruence, the basis for a working relationship.

Theoretical and experiential influences

This particular piece of work was structured and informed by a number of theoretical influences. I see it as underpinned by two significant perspectives: systems thinking and a task-centred approach.

Systems thinking

The work of Ann Hartman (1979) and Adele Holman (1983) in the United States has contributed very constructively to the application of systems thinking in work with prospective adopters. The insights afforded through viewing "the family as a transactional system, in constant interchange with its environment and developing through time" are rich indeed. An image which has remained with me from Virginia Satir's (1972) writing is that of the family mobile, each part intrinsically linked, with any movement or change reverberating throughout.

I think this approach is immensely valuable for a number of reasons. 'Thinking families', as Dr Eia Asen (1995) points out, yields data. The family is the major source of support and stress. The systemic perspective enhances the values of partnership and empowerment. The work can be an open, shared experience, enabling families to discover new insights and connections, rather than to be informed by 'the expert'. Viewing the family as an homeostatic system which will be impacted on by the addition of a newcomer is a good basis for considering what accommodation is going to be necessary to create a new balance.

The systemic approach also models a useful and constructive perspective for families. Those who can look at their total system for insight and understanding will have a much richer basis from which to approach issues and concerns post-placement. Emotionally damaged children make perfect scapegoats and are only too eager to take on the role of the 'villain of the piece'. With a systemic perspective the family can work towards changes in parents' behaviour, sibling roles, family priorities – rather than falling into the trap of seeking someone to 'fix' the child.

Task-centred approach

The second major influence is a task-orientated perspective which leans heavily on adult learning theory. Again, I see this as highly compatible with the underlying principles of partnership and empowerment, and indeed with systemic thinking. There are a number of clearly identified tasks which adoptive parents take on with their new role. David Kirk (1984) focuses on the twin tasks of acknowledging difference while creating a real sense of belonging. This approach helps families come to understand the components of their demanding role, see where these demands fit with their family, and decide for themselves with their worker whether it is a road that they are ready to go down.

Attachment

Insights and tools from other perspectives have also been helpful. Attachment is a key issue in this work. This year I came across for the first time Mary Main's (1991) work in this area. She puts forward the view that parents' mental representations of their childhood experiences of attachment can determine their sensitivity to the child's attachment needs. This is clearly central to adoption practice. This perspective has been developed in the past by many people, including John Bowlby (1969).

The congruence, in terms of internal coherence and plausibility, of the parents' narratives concerning their own attachment history is what Mary Main focuses on. This seems to be a much more helpful approach to understanding parents' history than that afforded by a more pyscho-dynamic model. Good childhood attachment experiences are not essential prerequisites to good parenting, but rather the ability to be in touch with, acknowledge and make meaningful sense of these experiences.

Attribution theory

One of the main tasks facing adoptive parents is sharing the child's preadoptive experiences. An element in this is acknowledging and understanding the ambivalent and conflicting feelings which many adopters experience when thinking about birth families. This was a significant issue for Alan at the early stage of this work. I was able to gain some valuable insights from attribution theory in understanding where he was coming from and in supporting him towards a significant degree of resolution.

Attribution theory helps us think about how we form explanations and how we make sense of behaviours. In this instance it was a useful framework for thinking about how the applicant explained the actions and responses of birth parents to himself. Thinking in terms of 'attribution errors' alerted us to where he was under-estimating the influence of a number of interacting factors and over-estimating the degree of control over life choices and responses. Shaver's (1985) work around the attribution of blame helped me think about the complexity of how we reach judgements and to use these insights to support Alan in developing a more tolerant perspective.

Trauma and loss

Undoubtedly my experience of working with children and families in the adoption context has a tremendous influence on this piece of work. My understanding of the very particular needs of children who have experienced trauma and loss has been informed not only by the writings of such people as Claudia Jewett (1984) and Vera Fahlberg (1994), but also by my direct involvement with many children and their families over the years.

The experience of trauma in my own professional background is also an influence which I try, with varying degrees of success, to be in touch with and to acknowledge. Within the context of this particular piece of work I was keenly aware that my only experience of disruption in adoption was a situation where the unmet needs of a birth child played a key role. The needs of Conor and Joanne in this family were quite rightly high on everyone's agenda, while I was aware that the meaning for me was informed by more painful experiences.

Process of the work

Over a six-month period I met with Alan, Melissa, Conor and Joanne fortnightly in their home. I also met with Alan and Melissa without the children, and had meetings with each individually. In reviewing the process I will look in some detail at two sessions and then at a recurring theme and how we worked with it.

As mentioned previously, the dual tasks of assessment and preparation were present throughout. I borrowed 'tools' from family therapy and systems thinking in structuring the work. Dynamic tools such as the ecomap and the genogram encouraged openness, trust and collaboration during the initial stages. I felt these were also very useful in engaging the children.

Session I

I planned this initial session around the ecomap, seeing it as expressing many of the values underpinning the work. Observing the process became for me at least as, if not more important than, the material which emerged (see ecomap, Figure 2).

When we got to work with a large sheet of paper and pens, all except Conor were immediately engaged. He had been asked to turn off the TV and was 'in a huff'. Alan acknowledged how Conor was feeling but remained firm, and went on using humour and exaggeration to diffuse feelings. He soon had Conor tucked in beside him and eager to join in.

As we got on with mapping I was able to share my observations and some hypotheses with the family, and use these for further exploration. I noticed that individual friends and activities were very much in place and encouraged. I could see this degree of openness around boundaries with the 'outside' world working well with another child. A great respect and value for the individual emerged here.

Figure 2: Ecomap

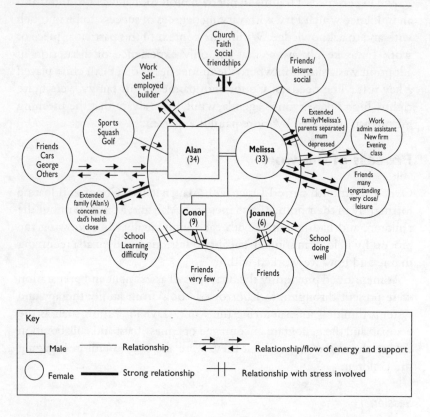

The map was also very useful in highlighting where the potential stresses lay: Alan's job, Melissa's parents and Conor's school work. We were able to examine each of these and flag up areas for exploration. The very strong supportive connections which the family had were also clear.

When we looked together at the completed map Alan and Melissa were able to think about what changes would be necessary to accommodate a newcomer. Melissa did not plan to continue working and would review this as attachments developed. We were able to look at the important and supportive links for her with friends and how these could be maintained.

Alan spoke of his weekends changing. He felt he was an involved, 'hands-on' dad, but thought that he would approach his parenting more consciously, with the need for time and space for everyone. Conor and Joanne joined in, thinking about strategies for organising family life to run more smoothly. Alan and Melissa listened and affirmed the helpful nature of their suggestions, while also saying that it was important that they had time to play and be with their friends.

Two of the particular issues which emerged from the map highlighted a number of points. One was the value and respect for children. As we mapped, Conor and Joanne were listened to, validated, and seen as individual young people who were developing and learning all the time. Melissa and Alan spoke of the concerns Conor was presenting at school. They included him very sensitively, encouraging him to express his opinions. Alan shared with Conor (not for the first time, I felt) his own difficulties at school.

Melissa spoke of the impact of her parents' separation and we were able to look at the changes in the lines of support. Melissa's mum used to visit each week and spend the day. Since her separation she had been very depressed and had withdrawn from the family. The map really helped in looking at the balance between stress and support, and in relating this to what Melissa and Alan were hoping to do in adding a new child to the family.

Thinking in terms of the tasks which would be undertaken with adoption, we were able to make connections with the emerging data. Many adoptive children have developmental delay and are experiencing difficulties at school. All of the family, especially Conor, could empathise with this and think what it would mean, and what they could put in place to help. Many children also come from situations where their parents are no longer together. Each of the family could see where they had experiences which they could use constructively to help them understand how an incoming child might be feeling.

Session 2

During this we constructed a genogram together. This was a powerful and emotive experience for all of us, and got in touch with some very deep feelings around loss and grief.

Before looking at this, I will consider some other issues that emerged. The connections with the extended family were very strong, particularly on Alan's side. In speaking of where they lived, what they were like and the degree of contact, it was clear how significant a role they played and what an impact any change in their circumstances had on this family, for example the paternal grandfather's heart attack and the maternal grandmother's depression. It was important to learn their views on the adoption application. In exploring these connections we could see there was a working balance between the support given to and that received from the wider family.

Joanne articulated the need to put on the genogram the babies who had died. Melissa had had four miscarriages since Joanne's birth, all around 17 to 19 weeks: this family was approaching adoption with a deep experience of loss in their lives, and it was important to explore this. I could see that these losses were acknowledged openly and supportively, and had been sensitively and significantly worked through. The family were in touch with their feelings but no longer in pain.

We were able to use this to look at other losses which are experienced by children separated from their birth families. Melissa and Alan were able to make the connection between their losses and their motivation in terms of adoption. They had mourned their babies, and did not see themselves as preoccupied with their loss in a way which would block their bonding with an adopted child.

I think we all found this an emotional and exhausting session. I found the ability of each of them to be sensitively aware of the other's position and to respect their differences very moving. More to the point, I was able to make a connection between the personal attributes and skills which they demonstrated and the need of adopted children for open, honest and age-appropriate discussion of sensitive and painful issues.

The genogram also served to highlight the pattern of relationships in the family. Conor had quite a significant position in the wider family, as the only boy among six grandchildren and the eldest. He 'lived in Alan's shoes' and also loved his grandfather's company. Melissa, Alan and Conor were able to make a connection between this observation and the question of the gender of an incoming child. It seemed important that I did not jump in and put some interpretation on this, but rather took time to facilitate their exploration of the issue.

This was very interesting in terms of their sensitivity to the different meanings gender would have for each of them. It emerged that the last baby who died had been a boy. They concluded that what was important was the need to be sensitive to the issue of gender, rather than feeling Conor needed to maintain his position as the only boy.

A wider issue

One of the tasks Alan and Melissa would need to take on was helping their adopted child integrate her or his life story with the story which would evolve in their family. How parents explain the child's life story to themselves will directly impact on how they help the child make sense of past experiences. In terms of the task-orientated aspect of this work, I saw Melissa and Alan as needing to reach some understanding of how children come to be permanently separated from their birth families.

Initially it seemed to me that Alan had a somewhat critical and blaming attitude to birth parents. Much research shows an association between compassion towards birth parents and successful placement. I needed to think about how I could enable and support him towards changing his perspective. My concern for him in parenting an adopted child while holding this view was openly shared. He was initially certain that his views would not impact on the adopted child, and was resistant to thinking he could come to a different view.

I think problems around blame and intolerance are particularly common when birth parents have been abusing their children. In exploring his views further I could see he was underestimating the complex interaction of a number of factors often present in situations where a child is abused. I needed to look at ways in which I could help Alan to a greater understanding of the damaging and stressful influences on parents which impact on their responsibility for their actions. I thought if this could happen he might see their culpability in a different light.

During this time I was aware of a number of issues impacting on our relationship. I felt concern about the 'power' issue and wondered whether he would feel he ought to move in his thinking in order to please me, and be seen to have the attributes of a 'good' adoptive dad: compassion and empathy for birth parents. Supervision was particularly important and necessary in exploring this issue. In one sense I could see where Alan was coming from: a very strong sense of individualism and a belief in free will. He was also a caring and compassionate man and I was hopeful that I could tap into this. He is very child-orientated and his sensitivity and empathy for children is immense. There was a real conflict for him in holding on to his feelings for the child and feeling any true empathy for the abusing parent.

In approaching work on this issue I put together some case material which focused on the fairly minute detail of the lives of birth parents who subsequently abused their children. This 'live' material helped us get to grips with the assumptions Alan held, and begin to unravel some of the distortions. I will look at this issue again in evaluating this work. We worked on this together in the sessions and Melissa and Alan did some 'homework'. Their task was to study a detailed history of a birth parent and think and rehearse how they would portray this to a child of Conor's age and a child of Joanne's age.

There were a number of opportunities created during the work to elaborate this issue. When Alan was very honestly speaking of an occasion when he had had to remove himself and put space between himself and one of the children because he experienced deep anger, he had relied very much on the support of Melissa in picking up the situation with the child. We were able to use this situation to look at 'what if' – you didn't have a supportive partner, had just had a very degrading experience claiming your social security benefit and were very depressed. It was important to use opportunities which naturally presented themselves to become further attuned to the complex position facing birth parents.

Evaluation of the work

Looking back to the principles underlying this piece of work, partnership and empowerment, I think we did succeed in building a working relationship together which is well rooted in these principles. I know from research and experience in this area that one of the crucial elements of preparation is the development of a relationship with the applicants which will be available to provide support and containment post-placement. I think the foundations were laid.

Thinking of the two essential tasks that were undertaken, assessment and preparing the family by helping them get in touch with aspects of their family functioning as it would relate to their role as adopters, the tools and insights borrowed from family therapy were very enabling. Enactment of the family dynamics and processes was much more valuable than relying on the family's narrative descriptions of how they worked together. It also was invaluable in underpinning the openness and transparency of the work. They were able to make connections and develop insights themselves, rather than me taking on the role of interpreter of the emerging data.

There were a number of instances of this. The genogram highlighted and facilitated exploration of the great losses the family had experienced, and allowed us to look at the meaning of these experiences and their central part in the motivation to adopt. This particular family map highlighted Conor's place in the family and his 'special' relationship with his dad and granddad. We were then able to use this insight to think about the meaning that the gender of an adopted child could have.

The process of completing this map and some others led to a very real enactment of how children are seen, valued, listened to and spoken with in this family. I was able to observe this and affirm its great value in relation to one of the key issues which concerns every adoptive parent, that of sharing in open, age-appropriate discussion the adopted child's life experiences. This was very empowering and affirming for the family. I think the process also reinforced their view of themselves as perhaps one of their own best resources in problem solving. As mentioned earlier, the systemic perspective can be a rich source of support post-placement, in looking at what everyone can do to address a concern.

The primary purpose of this work was not therapeutic intervention, but change did come about during it. As Alan and Melissa became more in touch with their family dynamics and more aware of the extra parenting issues they would take on as adoptive parents, they changed their assessment of the resource they could offer. At the outset of the application they were thinking in terms of two if not three children, and had no real 'limits' on what they could consider. At the end of the home study we were in agreement that one child would be right, and possibly two in a very particular circumstance, given the needs of the individual children.

The process of the work had highlighted not only the attachment needs of an incoming child, but also the need to be able to continue to meet the attachment needs of Conor and Joanne. They had been able to get in touch with the very particular needs of Conor especially, and to consider where his needs might possibly conflict with those of an incoming child.

The process helped in affirming a number of family norms congruent with the role of an adopting family. Tolerance of strong or ambivalent feelings is, in my experience, a very valuable attribute. In using an adaptation of Mary Main's adult attachment interview with Alan and Melissa, we were able to get in touch with the essence of their attachment relationships during childhood. Alan was able to think about the sense in which his parents were, as he said, "the bricks in his life", alongside what it meant to have a Victorian dad whose expectations and responses were at times very rigid.

Melissa got in touch with the very different relationships which she had with each of her parents, and, like Alan, became aware of how each parent contained positive and less positive attributes. Inevitably an adopted child, marked by conflict and confusion, is going to evoke powerful and ambivalent feelings. Alan and Melissa's ability to be in touch with past experiences which may be reawakened in this new relationship can only be a strength.

The ecomap helped identify a positive flexibility in parental roles within a more traditional gender role allocation. They each had particular roles but could easily take over one another's, especially when they could see signs of 'burnout' in the other. This ability will be a source of strength to them as adoptive parents.

The map also identified an open family system receptive to seeking and accepting support from a variety of sources. Evenings out separately and together, the occasional weekend away from the children, are seen as giving strength to the marital relationship. Maintaining outside interests and friendships restores perspective, relieves tension and refreshes everyone. They regard the appropriate support and involvement of those outside their family as a strength and an asset. We were able to recognise and affirm the value of this central family norm.

In evaluating this piece of work I can see where I could have had a more helpful perspective on a particular issue, and where I could have been more in touch with a power/gender issue which may have been impacting on what was happening. As I mentioned earlier, I felt quite early on that Alan was expressing feelings about abusive and neglecting birth parents that seemed to attribute a significant degree of blame. I was able to share my observations and my hypotheses around the problems I thought could follow from this perspective.

I structured my intervention around helping Alan gain a deeper understanding of the minutiae of the lives of birth parents, hoping he would then be able to get in touch with the complex web of circumstances and life experiences which were often beyond their control and determination. To a significant extent I think this intervention was successful in moving and changing his perspective but I now question whether I emphasised this issue too much, to the extent that I did not leave space to acknowledge the complex mixture of feelings towards birth parents which many adopters experience.

I think on reflection I put too much pressure on Alan to hold a compassionate and sympathetic stance. It would have been more helpful to emphasise the mixture of conflicting feelings he was experiencing, and to give more permission to express the negatives. Reflecting more on this issue, I have realised that if he is denied the opportunity to be in touch with and express the whole range of his feelings, how can he be open and responsive to the confused and ambivalent feelings which his adopted child may experience? The post-adoption centre in their work have looked at where 'glossing over' negative feelings in work with children can create an idealised and unreal picture of birth parents, which makes it very difficult for children to accept separation from this 'good' parent.

Much of the concern which arises early in this type of work is around disabusing prospective adopters of the idea that we have some sort of 'normative' family in mind, against whom they are being measured. We try hard to create space in which they can let go of the need to expend great energy on 'impression management' and providing the right answers. I think there is a sense in which the way I worked with the family on this particular issue may have undermined some of the work which was done around openness and empowerment. I also think there was a gender/power issue impacting on the developing relationship between myself and Alan which I was in touch with at a certain level, but not sufficiently to recognise the part it may have placed in creating resistance.

Does Alan feel I was telling him what to think, and where does this fit with feelings he may have of not being comfortably 'in control' of the process of their application? I was reminded of a discussion we had of his early attachments, when he described his dad as very rigid and dogmatic, saying "If he changed his mind he would never let on!" Might there be echoes of that sentiment in operation here? I can now see I did not pay sufficient attention to these questions. Had I done so I may have approached this issue and any resistance I perceived in a different manner.

As this is in a sense a mid-way evaluation, with the next step being presentation to the agency's panel with the recommendation to approve their application, I know that I can go back to the family and create an opportunity to explore these concerns more sensitively and constructively.

The Drays: Breaking the pattern of reactive behaviour

Stephen Kitchman

Position at the outset of the work

This work is set within the context of assessing and working with a family. I shall first make reference to background information before outlining the work undertaken and the aims. I shall then give an analysis of the work and discuss the learning I achieved.

The Drays are a relatively large family with six children (see genogram, Figure 1). They are white, working class and see themselves as indigenous to the East End of London. At the time of intervention the parents were married to each other and had lived together for 12 years. Both parents have large extended families who live throughout London, although there was reportedly little contact with them.

Initial social services assistance, for financial support, had been sought by the family two years after the birth of their first child Sarah. The file had been generally open throughout the 11 years since then. Before this, both parents had been 'looked after' in the care of the local authority, following rejection by their respective families in their early teens, although these case files had been destroyed.

At the point of allocation my role as prescribed by the transfer summary was 'to assess the need for and ... input family support as appropriate'. I was told that this case would not be too taxing and probably short term; which seemed a contradiction given the volume of case files. The rationale for my involvement seemed to be a reaction to the family's continuous presentations for support to an overburdened duty service.

Figure 1: Genogram

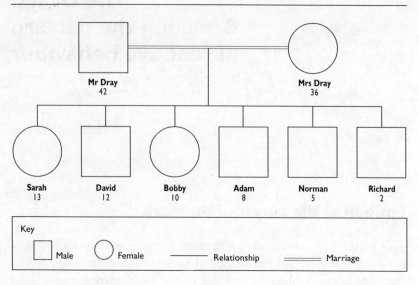

I began this work by creating space to read the case files. As with the initial referral, the files seemed to have been held open by the parents' persistent demands on social services for support, as opposed to statutory requirements. None of the children had ever been 'looked after' under the Children Act (1989) or previous childcare legislation. There had, however, been some instances of concern relating to Adam's suspected failure to thrive in 1989, and possible cigarette burns on Norman in 1993; both were recorded under the heading of 'no further action.' More recent incidents up to the end of my involvement included referrals from the GP and schools raising issues of neglect, injury and child protection.

Assessment of the situation

For my first visit, I requested that both parents be present and arranged to call at a time when the children would also be there. I saw this primarily as an introductory visit, and felt the children's presence would give me some insight into what the household might normally be like. I also felt that for the children to meet me might allay any fears of the unknown, or why a social worker was visiting

The family lived in a dilapidated four-storey town house. The inside was very dirty, with a strong odour from cat litter, broken furniture, overflowing rubbish bins, filthy kitchen and bathrooms, curtainless bedrooms; the garden was severely overgrown. Both parents were present on my arrival and two children raced up the stairs. In the lounge Richard lay asleep on the settee and did not stir; Adam sat on the other end of the settee. After introductions I asked how they saw their needs. Mrs Dray apologised for the state of the house, saying she hadn't had time to clean and we discussed this. She then continued to recount the need for children's clothing, furniture, help with the housing department, a nursery place for Richard and help organising the home.

Many of these requests fell within the remit of a family support officer, to whom the family and myself agreed a referral should be made. I asked to be introduced to the rest of the family and duly met Sarah, David, Bobby and Norman. For the first time the father spoke and said, "We'll need some help with this one as well", pointing to David. The mother immediately interjected "Leave him alone" in a fierce tone, and the father was silenced. I agreed to discuss David's needs further on my next visit.

On leaving the house my initial thoughts were pleasure at being able to breathe fresh air again and the desperate need for the house to be cleaned. Despite having six children neither parent worked, and so I believed both should be involved with cleaning the house. It was positive that the mother was aware of the need for cleaning but attention was still needed in this area. I was also aware that the father had distanced himself from this meeting and had been there only 'in body'. He had been the first one to make reference to the children but had effectively been silenced.

As much of my attention had focused on the mother, this seemed somewhat unfair, placing all responsibility on her, and despite unresolved questions about the family dynamics I felt that greater emphasis should be placed on the father's responsibility, and indeed he may have been responsible for undermining the mother. I was aware of gender and the danger of colluding with stereotypes of the female partner being responsible for childcare and domestic chores, giving the male partner no ownership of these concerns.

Process of the work

Prior to my next visit the father arrived unannounced at my office. He was extremely vocal and said that there were problems at home with his son David's behaviour, for example smoking, not coming in on time and swearing. Mr Dray felt that his wife always defended David whatever he did, and commented "Can you see what I have to put up with...." I responded that I could not as I did not know his family well enough, and suggested that we discuss his concerns when his wife was also present. He said he would try but there wasn't much point as his wife wouldn't listen. Then he advised me to be careful of giving his wife any payment, as she would often spend the money on herself.

I felt that Mr Dray had been strongly seeking collusion and validation for his feelings. This was possibly increased by our shared gender. There was also a certain childishness, which he presented in his refusal to talk when his wife was there, although I recognised that when he had spoken he had been stopped. I wondered what the effect on his wife might be, given that she knew he had come to see me. In view of this, I was pleased that the family support officer was female and hoped that this might encourage Mrs Dray, and allow me to challenge Mr Dray as appropriate, as well as allowing me to answer some of the questions I was forming.

My next visit to the family was with the family support officer. Mr Dray was extremely pleased to see us and chatted readily. There were some improvements to the house which he was eager to show us. We then sat down to negotiate a planned package of support from the family support officer. Given the great practical support that the family had previously had without change, their commitment and involvement would be needed. To express this clearly and give structure to the family support officer's role, a written agreement was made (Box 1). (For a fuller discussion of the uses and limitations of written agreements see Preston Shoot, 1994.)

Box 1: Contract of agreement

Between Mr and Mrs Dray, J.A. (Family Support Officer) and Steve Kitchman (Social Worker).

A new written agreement was drawn up between the above parties on......... The previous agreement lapsed due to the illness of the previous family support officer. The purpose of this agreement is to assist Mr and Mrs Dray with their parenting abilities, help make the home safe and hygienic, and assist with budgeting and routines.

The agreement is as follows:

1. Family Support Officer (FSO) to become involved to offer assistance to the family.

2. Social Worker (SW) to be allocated short term to oversee help to the family.

3. FSO will visit for a four-week period, the onset of this involvement to commence on...........

4. Both parents should attend all of FSO's meetings.

5. Appointments should be kept by all parties, unless emergencies arise about

6. FSO will explore what children's clothing and furniture are needed and what help is available.

7. Social services will fund stair gates. Mr and Mrs Dray to obtain cost and arrange fitting.

8. FSO and Mr and Mrs Dray to discuss after school provision for the children, eg Quest.

9. FSO to discuss budgeting and appropriate help with Mr and Mrs Dray.

10. Mrs Dray to obtain a notebook to record all incoming/outgoing finances.

11. Mr and Mrs Dray to provide information on finances and how they spend the money.

12. Mr and Mrs Dray and FSO to discuss safety and hygiene within the home and help available with this.

13. FSO will explore what holiday trips/provision may be available for the children.

14. No further finance will be given without planned agreement.

15. FSO and SW to explore what nursery provision may be available for Richard.

16. Mr and Mrs Dray and FSO to work on assertiveness about friends and allowing people to stay.

17. FSO will assist with liaising with the housing department regarding essential repairs.

18. Mr and Mrs Dray to focus on always knowing David's whereabouts to ensure his safety.

19. The above and future social work involvement will be discussed at a review on.........

This was useful in stipulating what both parties would do and also included Mr Dray, although towards the end of this meeting he again withdrew. A review meeting was set to oversee progress and any changes necessary to the plan. As case notes indicated some previous confusions over plans, a task-centred approach for our involvement seemed most appropriate. Much of this visit dealt with practical matters, and to increase the focus on the children's needs another date was set.

Within the week Mrs Dray called in at the office, unannounced. She said that her husband drank too much and had used their Income Support at the pub. She said that when he drank he was verbally abusive and the children were worried by this. We discussed this in-depth and what she might want to do about the situation. She said she hated him but at the end of the day he was the children's father and she would stay. Later that week Mr Dray again came to the office concerned at what his wife had said; at the same time Mrs Dray telephoned to tell Mr Dray "not to bother to come home".

A subsequent meeting was arranged with the parents to look at their difficulties. To both parents I put the concerns of the other and asked 'Is this how you want things to be?' Initially both said 'Yes' which surprised me, but later they were able to agree that they did wish change but were unsure how to achieve this. I agreed a referral to the local child and family consultation service for assessment of their therapeutic needs and exploration of how they were meeting their children's needs.

A referral was made, although the service needed some persuasion to accept this as the family had previously been referred, and their ability to use therapeutic assistance had been questioned. Subsequently contact was made with several of the children's schools. All of the children had special educational needs. There were certainly worries about David's behaviour at school and problems controlling this. Sarah was withdrawn at school, as were Bobby and Adam. There were general hygiene concerns and Sarah was teased due to her poor clothing. Teachers had 'gut' worries about the children, although these were non-specific.

In view of the above I agreed with my supervisor to approach the family to request a child-focused piece of work with each individual child. The rationale for this was that within the chaos of the family it was difficult to get a clear sight of the children's individual needs. Indeed much of the work had been overwhelmed by the parents' needs. Given their parents needs I wondered how much the children's needs could be met. This view is upheld by many of the child abuse inquiry reports, which document how the parents' needs overwhelmed the social workers.

The reports also highlight the large number of previous injuries to, or concerns around, the children as a significant factor (DoH, 1991a).

I thought that the children were now meeting their developmental milestones but seemed emotionally bereft. A large scale NSPCC study (Williams, 1996) indicates that 50% of the sample abused as children suffered without speaking out. Despite this many felt that they were giving out signs that could have been picked up by those around them. Additional research (Kitchman, 1996) gives weight to the need to speak to children about their experience.

Following my return from annual leave, I made a visit to discuss these sessions with the parents, but there was no reply. I had also hoped to discuss the work with the children and had planned to use direct work, for example, ecomaps (DoH, 1988), to talk about their support networks and experience. I later learned that David was in hospital with serious burns from experimenting with lighter fluid. Due to the severity and frequency of injuries, enquiries under Section 44 of the Children Act (1989) were made with the police child protection team.

David recovered but before I could speak with him I received a call from Mrs Dray to say that the family had moved to the South Coast. Investigations were transferred to the appropriate authority. Another message was received to say that Mr Dray had moved to Leicestershire permanently, following a recent relationship with another woman.

Evaluation and discussion of the learning

This account deliberately emphasises my feelings as a worker, with events constantly making me wonder what would happen next. As well as this, it was frustrating that the family were not able to utilise the input given and moved before my plans for a child-centred approach could progress further. Physical conditions had improved slightly. Obviously there are many subjective variations about what constitutes appropriate standards but there was consensus even within the family that levels were too low. It is interesting to note the original catch-all remit of 'providing family support', and how my focus had developed through involvement. The fine line between service under Part III of the Children Act (1989) and more protective measures is again highlighted.

There is great scope for analysis in this family. From a systemic approach we can see the importance of David in the family, especially as a "marital distance regulator" (Reder and Duncan, 1995, p 41). Here, with the parents continually arguing over the boundaries with David, this served to keep them apart and prevented them from addressing other relationship concerns. For the parents, the children were something for them to battle over.

From my knowledge of and contact with the children, I would suspect attachment problems. (For further discussion of indicators of attachment disorder, see Fahlberg, 1994.) Indicators could be identified in David's inability to contain his frustration in school, and his siblings' withdrawn behaviour and isolation from their peers.

This might stem from the parents' own attachment disorder and their own unmet needs within the care system, for, as Bowlby states, "Parents' mental representations of their childhood experiences with attachment relationships ... are thought to determine their child's attachment needs and behaviour, and to influence the quality of parenting a child receives" (quoted in Reder and Lucey, 1995, p 137). Indeed much of the parenting the Drays were offering could be seen as neglectful, coupled with emotional unavailability and unresponsiveness. (For further indicators of neglect/emotional abuse, see Glaser, 1995.)

In view of the long history of social services involvement and knowledge of the family, a continuing response of giving financial support seems inadequate. Despite case recording of the parents' low abilities, they had become one of the best financed families in the area. Organisationally I feel that social services unconsciously went some way to supporting the situation. As the parents presented as needy and grateful for past help, social services became almost a parent.

Parallels to this pattern may be seen in the Bridge Report into the death of Paul (Bridge Child Care Consultancy Service, 1995). There is pressure for the worker to collude and continue. Mattinson and Sinclair (1979) refer to this as the "reflection process" (p 55). Within the organisation some workers referred to this family as "the dirty Drays". This and other assumptions about this family led to some level of acceptance of their behaviour, believing "that's just the way they are". This may be seen as an 'organisational defence', halting intervention.

The family's premature move also sabotaged opportunities to review the written agreement and progress made. Here I feel that we had been clear about what improvements needed to be made and hope that social services in their new area will continue to monitor these. If standards do not improve, the conflict between the "organisational defences" (Mattinson and Sinclair, 1979, p 58) and the need for further action might become evident.

I was surprised at Mr Dray leaving the family, as despite both parents' avowed mutual hostility the situation had lasted for some time. This is highlighted in the psychoanalytic notion of splitting (Mattinson and

Sinclair, 1979, p 54), where people can simultaneously hold strong conflicting feelings about one another. Both parents consciously rejected each other, but unconscious yearning was apparent if one of them was absent. I believe without the affair Mr Dray would probably not have left, as he needs someone to be available to fill his emotional void, and without a partner or children there may not seem much else.

I felt I had been quite structured in my intervention, although I can see how easy it can be to be drawn into the sense of family mayhem. Acknowledging the impossibility and undesirability of complete detachment, good planning and interagency communication goes some way, I feel, to assisting objectivity.

Although the ending of this piece of work was premature and unsatisfactory, I hope that it may be continued by the new social services department with which I have fully communicated. I have been reminded of the complexity of family work and the need for continuous reflection on my role as a social worker within this context. Input needs to be reviewed accordingly, so that the focus on the child is not lost. I feel that this has been a salient learning point for working with families with such a high level of chaos. If the agencies involved seem swamped by the chaos we must again explore the impact of this on the child.

The Reids:
Putting boundaries in place

Michael Atkinson

Background information

The Reid family first became known to social services in 1992. Darren, the father, presented himself unexpectedly at a local family centre asking for advice and guidance after physically assaulting his son, Paul. The assault was so severe that Christine fled with Paul and their daughter, Kay, to safe accommodation.

At the time they were living in a nearby county authority where the social services department conferenced the family and placed Paul's name on the child protection register, under the category of physical abuse. However, after a three-month period the family reunited and moved back to the London borough.

Darren was charged with actual bodily harm in relation to Paul and sentenced to two years probation. This made Darren a schedule one offender. Probation and social services subsequently offered the family packages of treatment and assessment. Darren was referred to a clinic and completed attendance at an 'anger management group'. However, Darren was not particularly satisfied with the effectiveness of the groupwork. Although his personal assessment was paradoxical (he claimed that he did the majority of talking and had not received any advice; however, he also felt that the facilitators wanted to change his entire personality), Darren did engage well when offered individual work and achieved some change.

For the same period Christine attended a 'childcare management group' as she was experiencing behaviour problems in relation to Paul. Christine gained a lot of support from the group, but the facilitators were concerned about her attachment with Paul. Ironically the children's group workers were more concerned about the behaviour and development of Kay.

During the course of the group Christine shared that Darren had been sexually abused as a child and linked this to his rages. This disclosure posed an ethical dilemma for one of the group facilitators, as he was also undertaking the individual work with Darren. Unable to betray Christine's confidence, yet uncomfortable about working with secrets, he repeatedly tried to tease this disclosure out. Darren resisted.

Paul received some direct work in order to explore his perception of events and the effects of the 'attachment problems'. Paul responded well to this, and particularly to the use of fantasy games. However, despite this, Paul continued to get into serious trouble at school and had real problems with making and maintaining relationships. Paul was deregistered early in 1994.

Meanwhile, as Kay was displaying increasingly bizarre behaviour, the family were allocated a day care place at the children's centre I manage. Here the workers became concerned about Kay's behaviour and development and helped instigate an educational assessment (statement). We worked with the family for 18 months; during this time I built a trusting relationship with both Christine and Darren and had some contact with Paul. Kay eventually left the centre and moved to specialist provision for autistic children. Christine was pregnant at the time that Kay left.

Position at the outset of the work

In April Darren contacted one of the borough's family centres. He said that Paul, now aged nine, was still having problems at school and had been excluded on a number of occasions. He also emphasised that he was concerned about Christine's relationship with Paul. He felt that Paul did not 'respect' Christine and said he was fed up with having to 'control' Paul. He asked if the centre could help Christine. The family were also considering the option of Paul leaving home and boarding at a school out of London. The education department had discussed this with them and agreed to arrange it if they wanted.

The referral was supported by the allocated social worker and occupational therapist. Both these professionals were primarily involved because Kay was a 'child in need'. However, they felt that the family's management of Paul was impacting on the quality of care offered to Kay and their one-year-old daughter Kelly.

My assessment of the situation and negotiation of my intervention

My initial assessment of the family situation (and the course of my intervention) fell into a number of themes. Initially I took the following issues into account:

- the quality of attachment between Paul and Christine (Bowlby, 1969);
- Darren's role in the family system and his responsibility;
- that the family had previously experienced social services involvement as part of an assessment process;
- Darren is a schedule one offender with a history of violence; I also knew that Darren had been sexually abused and sensed that there could be a link between this trauma and his 'rages', that seemed consistent with dissociated behaviour (Van der Kelk, 1987);
- Paul was displaying troubled behaviour and the family were considering placing him in a boarding school.

I needed to consider my previous involvement with the family and their perception of me as an 'expert' in childcare matters. I felt that there could be a possibility of me being forced into an 'advice giving' role concerning issues of 'child guidance', rather than being allowed to work therapeutically with the family as a system.

Prior to my intervention, however, I felt that it was important to arrange a network meeting. The purpose of this was to interview the family and professional system involved, in order to formulate concrete boundaries to my therapeutic intervention (Asen, 1996).

I invited Christine, Darren, the allocated social worker and occupational therapist. I explained the purpose of the meeting and felt that it was important, not least to the professionals involved, to emphasise that that it was the family that had referred themselves to the family centre. This also gave me an early opportunity to explore both Darren's and Christine's perception of 'the problem'. I stressed my commitment to openness and the practice of working within agreed ground rules (see Box 1) and open recording (see Box 2).

At the meeting I also acknowledged how my role would be different. Interestingly this did not seem to be an issue for Christine and Darren, who felt that it would allow them to feel more relaxed. However, the occupational therapist repeatedly returned to the issue of 'poor child guidance' as the key to the problem. On these occasions she tended to imply that I was an 'expert' in the field.

During the course of the meeting Darren and Christine enacted a 'complementary relationship' (Burnham, 1986), with Darren adopting the 'one-up' position and Christine the 'one-down'. An excerpt:

Darren: "I'm the only one Paul listens to and I'm sick of it!"

Christine: "He never listens to me and I don't know what to do about it.' [looks at Darren]

They both appeared to be particularly entrenched in their relative positions.

What was also happening at this particular juncture was that the occupational therapist was being overtly sympathetic to Darren and repeatedly patronising to Christine. This 'mirroring' (Mattinson, 1992) or 'projective identification', where a professional identifies with one side of the family and acts out the family conflicts (Reder et al, 1993), seemed familiar to the family and made them more stuck. Despite this pattern both Darren and Christine responded honestly to circular questions.

Towards the end of the meeting both parents had added useful information to the fairly one dimensional referral about helping Christine manage Paul. The disclosures and developments I found particularly useful in my assessment of the situation were as follows:

• Christine said that there were times when she really wanted to show Paul that she loved him, but often she felt 'repulsed' by the physical closeness; she also said that she could remember her mother 'shuddering' in the same way when she tried to cuddle her as a little girl;

• Christine said that Paul often reminded her of Darren; with some probing she said this was related to the power Paul held over her;

• Darren acknowledged that the difficulties in the family did involve him and agreed to be involved in future sessions.

We agreed to focus on:

• how Paul can be physically and emotionally close to Christine in a comfortable way;

• moving away from blame and rigid positions of right and wrong.

Box 1: Working agreement

1. Personal safety

    Any disagreement or conflicts will be dealt with in the session. Individuals must feel confident to raise issues without worrying about their personal safety at home.

2. Individual responsibility

    Each family member should try and take individual responsibility for working towards agreed changes.

3. Confidentiality

    The discussions in the group will be confidential.

4. Attendance

    Everybody will make an effort to attend the sessions. If, for any reason, this is not possible as much notice as possible will be given.

5. Regularity

    The meetings will be on at least a fortnightly basis, initially for six sessions.

Box 2 (a): First meeting agenda

*   Working agreement/contract
*   Safety
*   Individual responsibility
*   Confidentiality
*   Accountability
*   Attendance
*   Regularity
*   Aims of the work
*   Hopes and feelings
*   What are we unhappy about/how can we change it?
*   Parameters
*   Safety for Paul
*   Power/who owns the power?
*   Acknowledgement of previous social service involvement (not an assessment): this will be a discussion/I will write up

- Ecograms: represent the people and things that are important to you; or three things Paul likes about Darren/Christine; three things they like about Paul?
- Next meeting

Box 2(b): Second meeting minutes

- Talked about a particular incident. Darren's violence towards Christine.
- Discussed impact on Paul (who said he heard what was happening).
- Talked about saying 'Sorry'. What does it mean? (Paul got upset and said 'Sorry is never enough for him'.)
- What do you want? Christine: "For it to be better between me and Paul." Paul: "For Mum to take me out sometimes and Darren to look after Kay and Kelly." Darren: "For Paul to listen to his mum."
- Common ground. Christine/Paul: quality of relationship. Darren: sharing control.
- We talked about 'making friends'.
- We all agreed to explore: Christine and Paul's relationship; moving away from blame.

Theories and experiences that have shaped my intervention

The approach I used reflected aspects of systemic thinking used in family therapy. This has been influenced by my own reading and training in systemic family therapy and greatly encouraged by the lectures of Eia Asen on the Goldsmiths course (Asen, 1996).

Systems theory

Although the variety of concepts and strategies I employed would be under the umbrella of 'systems theories', my approach does not reflect a particular camp. I felt that the working principles of hypothesising, circularity and neutrality (Palazzoli et al, 1980) would be particularly useful, given the complexities and 'stuckness' of this family. Testing hypotheses by circular questioning tends to create a dynamic environment that could encourage creativity and change in this family.

I felt that it was essential to acknowledge the gender and power dynamics in the family, given that:

- we were exploring a mother's relationship to her son, who she felt had too much power;
- Darren had a history of violence towards both Christine and Paul and appeared to use the threat of violence to gain control in the family;
- Christine already seemed to have a more healthy attachment to her two daughters, despite Kay's autism.

I aimed to incorporate some aspects of feminist thinking into my systemic practice. This is clearly more easily said than done. It also impacts on the role of the therapist who, according to the Milan ideal, keeps their values out of the interaction with the family. To an extent this required a shift in the application of key concepts, not least 'neutrality'.

To modify this concept I felt that I needed to explore with the less powerful the possibilities of increasing their power, while maintaining a view of the impact of this on the more powerful, in order to avoid a return to the status quo. Moreover, I needed to direct my attention to the family history with its myths, gender and other roles, and the social context in which the individual is shaped (Goldner et al, 1990).

Structural theory

I felt that aspects of structural theory were also relevant, given that:

- I had been presented with a specific problem and a request for help; there also seemed to be a commitment to change;
- there appeared to be 'disengagement' and also confusion or lack of clarity about the 'subsystem boundaries' (Minuchin, 1974);
- there were symptoms of problems in both the parents and sibling subsystems;
- a coalition had developed within the triadic relationship that was leading to Paul being 'scapegoated' (Haley, 1976).

I felt it would be useful to use 'enactment' to explore these areas. Enactment would allow me to observe the family members' verbal and non-verbal ways of signalling to each other, and to intensify some moments and prolong others. It would also give me a chance to probe and dictate alternative transactions (Minuchin and Fishman, 1981).

I also considered the family's stage in their 'life cycle' (Carter and McGoldrick, 1980). The family were clearly struggling with the developmental transitions of childrearing. I felt that this was complicated by Kay's special needs, which resulted in intensified stress, disruption and realignment. There also seemed to be a sense of the loss of a child.

As well as using the life cycle conceptually, I also tried to use the model to guide my interventions (Hughes et al, 1978; Haley, 1980). This involves four stages:

- engaging families so as to prepare them for the eventual effects of intervention;
- unbalancing the family, based on the idea that one of the causes of the difficulties is the family's rigid organisation and their thwarted attempts to progress developmentally; the intervention needs to be powerful enough to unbalance the system and so free it from its impasse;
- dealing with the consequences of change, given that it often produces some negative effects;
- disengaging, leaving the family functioning within its life cycle stage.

Attachment theory

Although systemic thinking formed the foundation of my work with the family, I also needed to acknowledge the influence of a number of other theories. Attachment theory (Bowlby, 1969) seemed a particularly important consideration, given the concerns Christine expressed about physical closeness with Paul who appeared insecurely attached, as did the notion of the 'positive interaction cycle' (Fahlberg, 1981a).

I was also particularly struck by Darren's accounts of his violent behaviour and subsequent memory lapses. A number of writers have described similar behaviour as 'dissociated' and linked it with childhood trauma, particularly child sexual abuse. Some also suggest that abuse may motivate the development of dissociated states as a defence against post-traumatic stress (Van der Kelk, 1987). This theoretical framework could allow me to explore any connection between Darren's behaviour and his childhood experiences.

Paul seemed to be displaying many of the characteristics of a child who is emotionally abused. He appeared to incorporate the acting on this in a self-fulfilling way (Bowlby, 1988). I was also mindful that there were elements of 'persistent negative misattribution' towards Paul and 'emotional unavailability' at least in relation to Christine (Glaser, 1995). I wanted to reflect some of these concerns back to the parents.

Lastly I felt I needed to address the risks that Paul may face as an emotionally needy child. I was concerned that Paul could be vulnerable to those who he turned to for support and be easily 'groomed' for sexual abuse. I used the time with the family to explore the parents' role as 'external inhibitors' and Paul's awareness of protecting himself (Finkelhor, 1984).

Process of the work

Darren's avoidance (burping and circular questioning)

As I mentioned earlier, before the initial family session I had organised a 'network meeting' where we had managed to agree on the parameters of the work, namely looking at Christine's relationship to Paul and Darren's influence. However, at the first meeting Darren wanted it to be clear to myself and other family members that he did not understand why he 'had to attend'. Interestingly he also adopted an ambiguous position of not wanting to be ignored. To this end he employed a variety of strategies. These ranged from interrupting or contradicting both Paul and Christine, to burping or breaking wind.

This posturing lasted for much of the first session, but subsided dramatically when questioning was reflected back to Darren, for instance 'Why do you think you are here?'; and even more so when triadic questions were posed, for instance 'Christine, does Darren's unwillingness to be here make it more difficult for you to say why you're here?'

The coalition (inquisition)

Once Darren became more engaged, the dynamics between father–mother–son changed dramatically. Darren and Christine formed a coalition, using the session to report one 'crime' after another. At each juncture I would suggest that Darren or Christine imagine, ask each other or ask Paul why these things were happening. Invariably when Paul offered reasons these were dismissed as 'excuses'.

Although I initially encouraged the family to 'enact' these interrogations, Paul seemed distressed and I felt it could be abusive to continue with this strategy. However, we did discuss how the family moved on after these incidents (my hypothesis being that they get stuck and accumulate evidence against Paul). Christine was able to say that there were times when she over-reacted, but that she always said 'Sorry'. At this point Paul said simply "When I say sorry, you say sorry's not enough!"

I felt that the relevance of this anecdote was not that it represented inequality between the partner/sibling subsystems, which could be justified or at least consistent with most families, but that the boundaries were confused and unclear. This shifted the family to focus on what Paul understands when he is being disciplined, rather than how the adults feel when Paul does something wrong.

Family circles (isolation and pets as friends)

This exercise proved to be a very powerful way for the family members to compare their internal and external worlds. Both Christine and Darren represented very isolated, nuclear family models. Darren's only external influence was football (see Figure 1). Christine only represented her sister-in-law outside her immediate family. This lead to a discussion around feelings of being trapped. Both parents reflected on the lack of support and resources to help with the care of Kay. They also spoke of the amount of time and energy that Kay required, and the effect on their relationship with each other and Paul. This obviously resonated with Paul who, experiencing this openness for the first time, was able to share his feelings of resentment.

Interestingly Paul asked to be separate from his parents while drawing his family circles. Paul's family circle was even more striking in its omissions. His only additions to the immediate family were two 'sonic' computer games which he had lost and three dogs. Under each dog Paul had carefully written 'Dead. I miss them'. This led to a discussion about what qualities we like in our friends and how we learn to make relationships.

This allowed the family to hypothesise themselves about Paul's attachment affecting his attachment to others. Paul's simple diagram formed the agenda for a couple of sessions, and it also introduced the notion of Paul's emotional vulnerability. In fact both Christine and Darren made this connection with little help from me. As Darren perceptively said, "If someone asks Paul to come and see his puppies, he's going to go, isn't he?"

At this point Darren was clearly in touch with issues of risk and protection and it was felt that we could have struck a nerve concerning his own abuse.

Figure 1: Darren's family circle

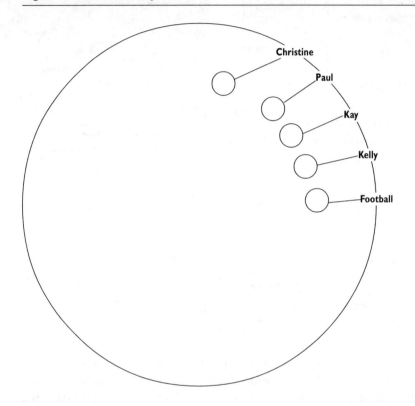

Genograms (favouritism and violence)

I knew from discussions with Christine and Darren that any discussion of family history would involve unpleasant, violent and abusive memories. For this reason I chose to exclude Paul from this session. Two very strong themes came out of the genogram exercise, representing different sides of the lineage, violence and favouritism (see Figure 2).

Darren described his father as an extremely violent man, who physically abused the children and Darren's mother. Darren was extremely protective of his mother at that time. His father was frequently in and out of the home. When asked if any of this history could have affected him, he was extremely resistant. At first he stressed that he was different, wanting to distance himself from his 'demon' father, but nevertheless he could make a number of connections between his father's relationship to his mother and his relationship with Christine. Christine was quick to echo this.

Figure 2: Genogram

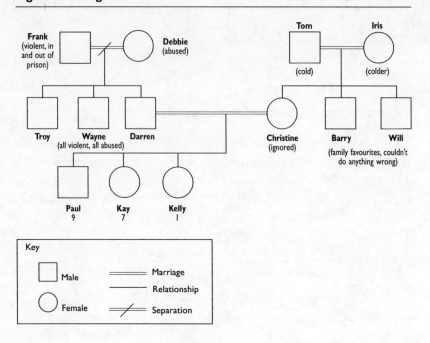

Key

Christine described her parents as being 'stable', but she said she never felt particularly close to them. Her two brothers were highly favoured and she still felt resentment about this. Unlike Darren, Christine was highly fatalistic about the long-term effects on her and Paul. On one level making these connections is healthy, but I felt that it was important to introduce the possibility of change and difference in family histories. We explored the difference in both families and discussed those who had 'escaped'.

Nearing the end

I became aware that all of the family members were becoming stronger individually. Christine appeared to be making the most ground. There also seemed to be an awareness of how one member could affect the other. Unfortunately Darren was unable to attend the most recent session as he has started working shifts as a fork lift truck driver. During the session Christine told me that Darren had in fact moved out and that she had been instrumental in this. I agreed to continue working with the family and continue to focus on Christine and Paul's relationship.

Darren did in fact arrive towards the end of the session to offer Christine a lift home. I sensed he wanted to use the session as 'marriage guidance', which I resisted. Work is still ongoing.

My evaluation of the intervention

Given the complexity of the dynamics, belief systems and history of this family, I am very encouraged by the success of the intervention. To gauge this most accurately I feel I need to refer to the negotiated purpose of the work, rather than hypothesise about many of the new issues raised by the family. The purpose at the outset was to focus on:

- Christine's attachment to Paul;
- the use of blame and avoidance;
- Darren's role in the family system.

Both Christine and Darren appear to have adopted a 'two-way traffic' approach to their interaction with Paul. During the course of the intervention it has been particularly effective to reflect the 'problems' back to the family. On one level this served to set parameters to our discussions. It also provided the family with a chance to reframe the nature of the problem. As with most problem definitions there tends to be some reference, either direct or obtuse, to its cause. What I have observed is a clear shift from linear to circular thinking. The family seem to analyse their problems in a more sophisticated way than simply A equalling B.

This circularity has allowed the family to shift from a model of blame (as they are all part of the problem). It also lead to a rethink, most notably by Darren, as to whose problems these are (as the problem is part of all of them). As a result Paul has been less marginalised and I have experienced some very 'warm' moments in the sessions. This change in atmosphere has been echoed by others involved with the family at home. The family themselves have expressed how useful the work has been, particularly the family circles exercise.

Despite this dramatic shift in the family I feel there are deep-rooted problems pertaining to both Christine and Darren, namely Darren's violent rages and Christine's 'gut feelings' of 'repulsions' towards Paul. I would question whether my work has addressed these areas satisfactorily. I will recommend to them both that they seek some help individually.

I know that Paul is presently in touch with the educational psychology service, and hope this will provide him with some individual space. I recently spoke to the field social worker to negotiate some extra support for the family regarding Kay. She is investigating both outreach and respite care packages.

What I have learnt and thoughts on how to develop this learning

This piece of work has allowed me to incorporate a huge amount of my learning into practice. One of my main problems has been to remain coherent with the family while my learning curve is on a vertical ascent. I will summarise the main themes of my learning. It has taught me or reaffirmed the following:

- The usefulness of having a theoretical structure underpinning the intervention, particularly the usefulness of 'systems thinking' when working with families.
- The importance of negotiation when working with families. This involves working with concrete problems and evaluating (and celebrating) change. I found the use of written agreements and open recording particularly useful.
- The impact of gender power when working with families, especially when there are issues of male violence and control. I benefitted from some enlightened reflective supervision, which focused my attention on the risks of mirroring, projection and unwitting collusion. An example of the latter was my use of a football analogy with Darren to represent a systems theory (although this did allow Darren to see a complex notion in concrete terms). I felt it was equally important not to compensate for this by conjuring up an artificial empathy with Christine to combat my own guilt and elevate my status as a 'new man'. When I next take on this sort of work I will carefully consider co-working with a woman colleague.
- The importance of supervision and a consultancy network. The supervision by my practice coordinator and consultancy with a family therapist were invaluable components to the work. Equally important was the learning and experience of the Goldsmiths tutorial group, coupled with lecturers working with live cases.
- How working actively with a family can stimulate one's own thinking and encourage future learning.
- How the family's confusion over the causes of their problems (or their avoidance) can impact emotionally on a child. This can involve

a child receiving confusing messages, or a definition of the problem/ solution inconsistent with their reality. I felt that Paul was often marginalised and I am concerned about the long-term affects of the misattribution of blame on him.

- The subversive effects of childhood trauma on adult behaviour and its impact on the interaction with their children and the outside world.

- How there is often a cost to change. Darren's most recent departure is one of many previous ones. However, I feel it is valid to infer that a power shift in the family enabled Christine to orchestrate this particular move.

- The safety, protection and ethical issues, when involving vulnerable members of a family. These issues became very real during some of the enactments and I subsequently decided to use different techniques when Paul was present. I was concerned that the sessions could lead to an escalation of violence, although, thankfully, I had no evidence of this. (Eia Asen spoke of the frequency of 'fights in the car park' in one of his lectures on the Goldsmiths course and this upped my anxiety level; Asen, 1996.) We addressed safety issues in a number of sessions and we had a written safety agreement; however, I feel I will need to consider this more carefully in the future.

The Green family: Work with a lone parent and her children

Patrick Lonergan

Position at the outset

The Green family are of white British origin. Ms Green, aged 33, is a lone parent with six children ranging in age from one to 12 years. They live in a three-bedroom ground-floor council flat in a tower block. At the beginning of this piece of work I had been working with this family for nearly three years. The focus had been the second eldest child Martin, aged 10 years, who had a poor relationship with his mother, which manifested itself in Martin presenting challenging behaviour.

An in-principle decision had been made by the joint education/ social services panel that a long-term placement should be sought for Martin at a 'therapeutic boarding school', with a view to rehabilitation after two years. As it was envisaged that this would be a lengthy process, it was agreed that Martin would be accommodated under Section 20 of the Children Act (1989) if Ms Green requested it. As his behaviour was putting the whole family at risk and had been for some months, a placement was found for him in a children's home in another borough.

While the focus of my work had been with Martin and his mother, I was aware that there were various issues in relation to all the children, but I felt I had not tackled them in a coherent and constructive manner. At the beginning of the year, I was feeling overwhelmed with the complexities of this case and I asked for a joint worker. Nobody suitable was available.

Doing the Goldsmiths course, however, and having the space – particularly in the three-week block at the beginning of it – gave me the impetus and confidence to tackle the case in a different way. For a genogram see Figure 1.

Figure 1: Genogram

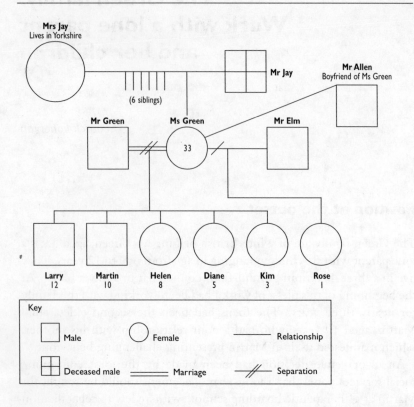

The resolve to take a fresh approach came when Ms Green told me her concerns about Kim, aged three, who, she told me, was not sleeping well, not eating, demanding a baby's bottle and generally regressing to 'babyish' behaviour. She wanted help with Kim's behaviour.

Assessment of the situation

In my time working with Ms Green I found that during the periods that Martin was 'accommodated', by and large she was able to manage the other five children, even though they presented different types of difficulties. The day-to-day demands of looking after a large family on Income Support frequently left her feeling overwhelmed and often left me feeling the same way, because she would frequently contact me by 'phone with her 'problems', and I did not have any simple answers for her, of course.

Ms Green's difficulties with Martin left her feeling a failure as a parent and she had poor self-esteem, all of which had been reinforced by the men in her previous two relationships. Furthermore, the various services that had been offered to help with Martin had failed to prevent him being 'accommodated' and separated from his family, so she felt the 'care system' had let her down as well. Also at times her own emotional needs were so great that it became difficult for her to focus on the needs of her own children.

Although she wanted Martin to be accommodated and to receive therapeutic help, like many parents in this situation she had tremendous guilt. While at this stage it was clear from my knowledge of the family that Martin had an insecure attachment to his mother, I was also worried about the quality of attachment in relation to the other children. As I said earlier, Ms Green seemed to be able to manage the other children but given that she had described Martin as a difficult child since he was two years old, what effect, I wondered, had this had on the functioning of the other children?

Martin's way of getting attention was through challenging behaviour. This was very successful and meant that Ms Green had very little time to devote to the needs of her other children. I knew that she had a tremendous commitment to her children, and that in the periods Martin had been accommodated she had always maintained contact and worked with social services or other agencies to the best of her abilities.

I embarked upon this piece of work, however, from the position that I felt Ms Green did have the ability to care adequately for her children, but these abilities needed to be nurtured and she had to be empowered as a parent to develop the confidence to improve her own parenting skills. Again, from my knowledge of her own childhood, I felt that she was in some respects replicating her own experience of childhood as one of a family of seven children.

Negotiation of my intervention

Before commencing the family work, I discussed with Ms Green my wish to work with her around issues concerning all the children, rather than focusing on individual children when 'problems' arose. We agreed, therefore, for the two of us to have a session together to map out her concerns and worries regarding all the children, so I avoided the situation where we just focused on Kim, while acknowledging we had to look at her behaviour.

At the same time, I should point out that Helen and Larry had had individual sessions with different workers outside the family home, which had been negotiated following a previous assessment by the local family centre. My focus was going to be on work within the home. Given that Martin was accommodated, I also had to continue working with him alongside this piece of work, so I was asking Ms Green to give a high level of commitment, as well as myself.

I negotiated with my manager extra time to undertake this work, as my caseload and time for cases is assessed under a workload management scheme operated within the department. The key principle of the Children Act (1989), partnership with families, was to the fore in this work. Because the children were on the borough's child protection register I had to inform other relevant professionals of my work as well, so we did not duplicate our involvement.

Influences, theoretical and/or experiential, that shaped my intervention

I decided to adopt a number of approaches to my practice, given the nature of the work I was undertaking, rather than a single method.

Systems theory

I thought it was important to draw ideas from systems theory and to look upon the family as a system, instead of focusing on individual parts, for example Martin's challenging behaviour. Asen and Tomson (1992) states that: "Family problems do not result from the behaviour of one person, but are connected to the way family members relate to each other. What each person does affects every other person and a chain reaction occurs" (p 4). With the Green family, I wanted to try and prevent what could become a snowballing of problems in relation to the other children.

Attachment theory

I thought that ideas based on attachment theory would provide useful pointers to assessing the individual children's relationships with their mother. Fahlberg describes attachments as "an affectionate bond between two individuals that endures through time and space and serves to join them emotionally" (Fahlberg, 1994, p 14). While none of the children presented the challenging behaviour that Martin exhibited, I did have some concerns about the emotional development of all of them.

At the same time, I was conscious of some of the criticisms of Bowlby's theories from a feminist perspective (Holmes, 1993). The main thrust is that Bowlby overstated his case regarding the effects on children of being separated from their mothers: the quality of substitute care is crucial, and children develop a hierarchy of attachment figures. I felt, however, that Bowlby's theories still had validity in evaluating levels of attachment. I believed that Martin's challenging behaviour stemmed from an insecure attachment, and I wanted to check out the quality of attachment in relation to the other children.

Child observation

In the early part of the Goldsmiths course I had carried out an observation on a two-year-old girl involving four one hour sessions over a period of a month. I found this a very useful exercise, and read some literature on the subject (Wilson, 1992). While it was not possible to do a similar exercise with the Green family, I did two mini-observation visits, which included all of the children, between the two sessions.

This proved valuable in assessing the interaction between Ms Green and her children; I planned to give her some feedback on my observations after the visits. As well as observing mother–child interaction I could also assess the children in terms of their development, particularly Rose, about whom there had been serious concerns in the past. I used the Mary Sheridan (Open University, 1990) charts on child development as a guideline.

Direct work with children

There were a number of ideas and methods I had learned about from sessions on the Goldsmiths course, which I felt I could use with Ms Green and the children to enable her to give her children some quality time.

The law

Section 17 of the Children Act (1989) outlines the duties of local authorities to children in need, in terms of promoting the welfare of children in their area. I felt very strongly that the emphasis in this work needed to be viewed from that perspective, and that I needed to examine what other services could be provided. Also central to my work was the philosophy of the Children Act, that children are best cared for in their own families, without resort to legal proceedings (White et al, 1990).

I chose this range of methods because I thought they were relevant to this practice situation; they suited my style of work and my approach to theoretical issues. From my previous knowledge of Ms Green I knew that while she actively sought help and guidance in relation to the difficulties with Martin, there had been difficulties for her in engaging with the family centre workers. I saw two principal reasons behind this:

- the approach to the family work was psychodynamic, which Ms Green had difficulty in relating to, and she found it fast paced;
- the practical difficulties of getting to the sessions on a regular basis when a number of the children had regular hospital appointments, for a variety of reasons.

I felt, therefore, that a different approach was needed, which was more directive and that took place in the home, so that practical obstacles were reduced as far as possible.

Anti-discriminatory practice

At the outset of this phase of my work with the Green family, I had directly discussed differences in terms of gender. In social work teaching and agencies, the words 'power', 'partnership' and 'acknowledging difference' are constantly used in discussion and reports. I see these concepts as integral to my work with the Green family. A useful definition of partnership for me is the following:

> The practice of working together with clients in such a way that all participants accord each other equal respect, and all clients are given as much say as possible in decisions that affect them. (Open University, 1990, p 5)

What both these definitions miss out, however, is the question of power, which is integral to fieldwork. In my work with the Green family and particularly Ms Green, I am conscious that there is a power imbalance in a number of areas. I am a white male worker for the local authority. I have to maintain a balance between working in partnership as defined above, but also being aware of having power invested in me to remove children, to determine the criteria for their return home to their families and to determine the criteria for what is 'good enough' parenting. In Ms Green's experience men had abused their power in their relationships with her. Her husband of 10 years had been violent towards her and left her with the prime responsibility for the children; Rose's father, with whom she shared a relationship for 20 months, had emotionally abused her, reinforcing her sense of failure as a parent.

Ms Green, having worked with me for the past three years, was aware of the power invested in me by the law. She had expressed to me her fears in the past about 'losing' not just Martin but all her children. They were all on the borough's child protection register, albeit because of Martin's behaviour. Martin had been accommodated in the past; she had attended a case conference, statutory reviews and numerous planning meetings with professionals, so when embarking on the family work she had an intimate knowledge of social services and how decisions were reached.

At the outset, I was aware of the delicate balance I was trying to achieve in my work. On the one hand, attempting to empower her as a woman, a lone parent, acknowledging her strengths. On the other, assessing her parenting skills and possibly moving from a position of viewing her children as 'children in need' as defined in Section 17 of the Children Act, to viewing them as children in need of protection and suffering significant harm as defined in Section 47 of the Act.

In working with families now, I am also aware of the intense media scrutiny of childcare social workers who can be seen as instantly removing children, and government attacks on lone-parent families, who are being perceived as inadequate, benefit scroungers and jumping the housing lists. In other words, as a drain on society's resources, which can only further damage the self-esteem of people like Ms Green. In one conversation, after her benefit was reduced because Martin is accommodated, she told me, "This government does not care whether I can feed my kids".

It is difficult, therefore, when working with families, many of whom are lone parents, to convince them that as social workers we are seeking to work in genuine partnership with them, and that our prime objective is to keep children within their birth families. I found O'Hagan and Dillenburger useful background reading in this area (1995). It was with all these factors in mind that I embarked upon my work. I found Margaret Adcock's (Adcock et al, 1988) diagrammatic representation of social workers in the context of society very useful.

Process of the work

In describing the work I am going to select what I believe were the key sessions, involving the children still living at home. Because of the complexity of the case I do not have the space to detail all the sessions.

I wish to concentrate principally on the setting up of the work and the sessions which I believe helped me assess the quality of attachment.

First session

I started by having two sessions in the office with Ms Green on her own. At the first, adapting the idea of family circles, I gave her a piece of flipchart paper and asked her to write down her name and the names of the children and, looking at each individual child, identify what are the current concerns for her as their mother. I remember before the session feeling a bit odd asking Ms Green to do this, given that I had been visiting her regularly for nearly three years, so I adapted an introduction from Asen (1996) and started off by saying, "I realise I know a lot about you, but at present there is so much going on with all the children, perhaps it would be useful if you could identify on paper what are the issues for you at the moment". While she was doing this I left the room and made her a cup of tea, as I did not want her to feel I was looking over her shoulder (see Figure 2 for details).

Figure 2: Ms Green's diagram of current concerns

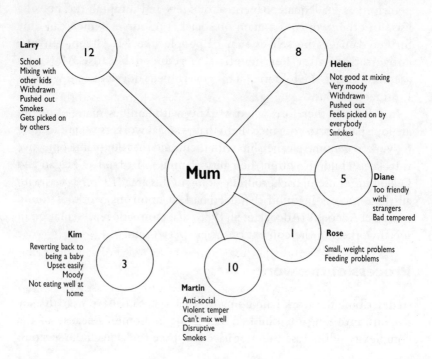

When she had finished we looked at what she had written. I wanted to see if, using systems theory, we could identify any patterns in terms of concerns affecting more than one child. I could point out that in the three eldest children, Larry, Martin and Helen, she had identified that none of them mixed well; two of the younger children, Kim and Rose, she identified as not eating properly (Rose was below the third centile); Larry and Helen she described as withdrawn, pushed out, getting picked on; Larry, Helen and Martin she believed were smoking.

I remember thinking that while I was aware of most of these concerns, seeing them all down on one piece of paper was quite startling; and how daunting the task would be of helping Ms Green with her concerns, as well as helping Martin to move on to a residential placement. I told her that after the second session the following week we would draw up a plan to tackle some of the issues.

Second session

In the second session, I asked Ms Green to write down who were the most important people in her life by drawing circles and to draw the circles in size according to their importance. What was striking about this was the paucity of people she wrote down (see Figure 3). I remarked upon this fact, and that she had not put down any members of her family except her mother (Ms Green is one of seven children). She told me how her mother had left her father when she was young and the only child she took with her was herself, as she was the baby. Her older siblings always resented this, she said, even though her mother returned again. I could sense the sadness in her voice when she said this.

I asked her to look at the diagrams she had drawn and, looking at her own children, if she saw any connection with her own childhood; at the same time I acknowledged with her this might bring up painful and sad feelings for her. She told me a little about her relationship with her ex-husband: how she had met him as a teenager and after getting married at 18 she had never gone out much because he would not allow her to, and as a result she never had any friends. It was only after he had left her that she started going out. A question I asked myself was whether Ms Green's childhood and adult experience of feeling isolated was being replicated in some of her own children.

These are only extracts from the sessions, but having asked Ms Green to describe her concerns I suggested to her that I would think about what she had written, and try and help her deal with some of them.

Figure 3: Ms Green's network

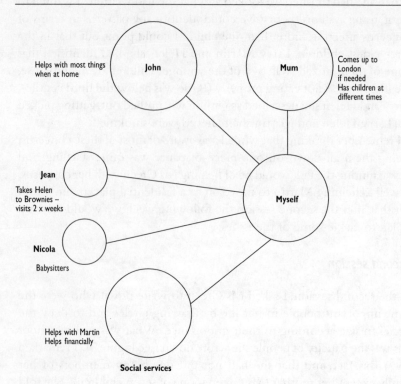

I already knew that Martin, aged 10, had an insecure attachment. Drawing on Bowlby's ideas I saw Martin as a child whose lack of security aroused a simultaneous wish to be close to his mother, and at the same time to punish her at the slightest hint of abandonment. While none of the other children exhibited similar behaviour, I did feel there were signs of poor attachment. My main concerns were around the following:

- initiating positive interaction with the children;
- responding to the younger children's overtures;
- with the older children, commenting on their positive behaviours as well as the negative.

This was based on my knowledge of the family and the concerns Ms Green herself had raised with me.

Observation visit

Given that I had got agreement with Ms Green to look at the needs of all the children, we agreed that I would do an observation visit in which I would observe her interaction with the children, and from that give her both positive and constructive criticism. I was waiting for an adverse reaction as this had been done before by the family centre, but it never came, which I felt was an indication of her commitment at this stage. I found the concept of using a 'family lens', described by Asen and Tomson (1992), useful in this process. Instead of focusing just on Kim, who had been clearly identified as the most problematic child at this stage, I was observing all the family members.

On that visit I was not a stranger to the children but, whenever they did approach me, I directed them away towards their mother or another sibling. Initially it was the three youngest children at home: Diane, five, Kim, nearly four, and Rose, nearly two. Larry and Helen came in around 4.15pm from school. I chose the time of day, 3.45pm–4.45pm, when the children came home from school, which Ms Green had found particularly problematic in the past. I sat in the living room where everybody usually sat, played, watched TV, and which adjoined the garden.

My main observations from the visit were that with the youngest three children, Ms Green largely sat by the door leading to the garden. From time to time the children would wander up to her and she would respond appropriately to their needs for attention, holding them on her lap or showing an interest in objects/toys they were showing her. In general, the children wandered from the living room down the corridor to another part of the flat, sometimes coming back with a toy, for example small children's tricycles, and wander off into the garden. Their play was quite separate and fights and arguments would ensue over toys, usually between Kim and Rose. Diane occupied herself with TV and lay on the floor watching it, turning around occasionally, drawing her mother's attention to what was on, and Ms Green would respond. Their concentration was fairly limited; hence, I thought, the tendency to wander around a lot.

Another pattern of behaviour was that Ms Green would shout at Kim and Rose from her chair when they were fighting, usually resulting in Rose bursting into tears. When they wandered into the garden she had to retrieve them a number of times, because the garden went from the side of the flat to the front and they wandered into the street. I remember being very uncomfortable when Kim and Rose went out of sight because

Ms Green had reported to me recently that Kim had wandered across the road to the playground.

Ms Green tended to sit issuing directions from her chair. When Larry and Helen came in they acknowledged my presence and Ms Green spoke to them both about their day at school and what they had been doing, which she did very appropriately. During the course of her conversation, which lasted ten minutes, the younger children, principally Kim and Rose, were also seeking her attention. What was striking was that there were now five children at home and only one adult. Ms Green by now was ignoring the attempts of Kim and Rose and Diane to catch her attention.

In discussing my observations with Ms Green I drew on my previous knowledge of the family and ideas I had learnt from the observational assessment of the two-year-old girl earlier in the year; and ideas on attachment from Bowlby (1988), Fahlberg (1994) and Katz et al (1994). I found Fahlberg's observation checklists very useful for assessing levels of attachment, and Bowlby's and Fahlberg's premise that providing physical and psychological safety and security is a basic parental task for carers of the young child; also Bowlby's assertion that two characteristics that strongly affect the level of attachment are the speed and intensity with which a mother responds to her child's crying, and the extent to which the mother herself initiates interaction with her child.

Session with Ms Green

I had a session with Ms Green on her own at the office to discuss my feedback from the observational visit and ideas for future sessions. I gave her the positive feedback on how she had engaged with Larry and Helen, and that by and large she had responded to the younger children when they had sought her attention. I commented that while the children did play, their concentration was not too good and that, if she perhaps engaged more actively with them, it might help keep their focus more on play, and stop them wandering off so often. I discussed the importance of routine for the children and creating a structure to their day with which they could become familiar, and at the same time meet some of their individual needs.

Given the feeding issues with the two youngest children she herself had identified, which were being monitored by the health visitor, I agreed to provide financial assistance through the Section 17 budget for a table and chairs. My child observation earlier in the year had identified teatime as an integral part of the sessions, and I had been struck by how enjoyable and relaxed this time was for the two-year-old girl, with lots of interaction between the mother and her child.

Ms Green was obviously pleased with this offer of practical assistance and we drew up a plan for developing a routine for the children after school, which revolved around spending quality time with them. For Rose this could be achieved during the daytime when she was at home on her own; for Larry and Helen we identified the best time as after the younger children had gone to bed. For Kim and Diane it was the period between returning home from school, up to and including bedtime. Bedtimes and mealtimes were identified as a key time for Kim, given her difficulties around sleeping and feeding.

I knew from previous visits that in the past four months there had been no dining table, so the older children ate on the floor and the younger ones wandered around with food in their hands, so clearly it was not a very good experience or structure, making it difficult for Ms Green to encourage Kim and Rose to eat. I acknowledged the burden and difficulties for her of managing five children at home and also maintaining her relationship with Martin, who was accommodated in a children's home 10 miles away in another part of London.

Further sessions

We planned a few sessions, therefore, when I would visit at different times, and bring along play materials which she could use with the children. I tried to bring along materials/toys which were not too expensive, as I was conscious that Ms Green was on Income Support and I wanted her to use these ideas and materials herself outside of our sessions, and be able to afford to buy them or similar materials/toys. Again I used the Section 17 budget, arguing that these were 'children in need'. I also wanted to do another mini-observation around teatime, so I could check out the mealtime routine. At that session the children did sit at the table, and were able to use cutlery appropriately. I encouraged Ms Green to sit with them. Kim and Rose both ate their meals. The structure clearly worked.

I saw play as a very important tool, not only for the development of the children but as a means by which Ms Green could develop more interaction with her children, and thereby increase the level of attachment, particularly in relation to the younger ones. I think Cattenach (1992) describes the importance of play very well when she says, "Play is the central experience for the child in helping her to make sense of the world around her, and her place in that world" (p 29). I shared this knowledge and concept with Ms Green.

Unfortunately these sessions were delayed because Martin kept absconding from his placement and over a two-week period he returned home four or five times. This caused major disruption to the household and he strongly resisted going back. These events often occurred in the evening, so it was the night duty social worker who returned him. It also negated any attempts at this stage to establish a routine for the children. I found another placement for Martin while we continued the search for a suitable long-term placement.

I acted as a 'mentor' in the sessions but observed as much as possible and encouraged Ms Green to actively participate. For various reasons I rarely managed to engage all five children, which was disappointing. It was usually Larry, the eldest, who was missing or came in part way through. I will elaborate on this later. Generally, the sessions were successful in that Ms Green did manage to engage with her children much more actively and intervene appropriately to stop arguments, without resorting to the shouting method she usually used when sitting apart from them. Three key sessions were playing with clay and water in the garden, playing with Duplo and constructing a house, and a drawing session including Kim and Diane doing wonderful life size drawings of themselves, which Ms Green put up on the wall and the back of a door. (Rose was absent for this one.)

For me these sessions were valuable because they showed me that when the children were given some structure and direction, they could play and enjoy activities together. Even though there were distractions with people calling at the house, the sessions were not severely disrupted, in contrast to my earlier observation session. The regular scenario of Ms Green talking at length about her day-to-day problems and the younger children wandering around a lot, appearing rather lost, was avoided. I did not have my usual anxiety of feeling that one of the younger ones had disappeared outside on to the street. I encouraged Ms Green to be in the garden herself so she could keep a closer eye on them, and the clay sessions took place in the garden. Overall, instead of the chaos I usually felt when visiting, I came away less anxious because the home situation seemed less chaotic, and more contained.

Obviously on these visits I did have to discuss day-to-day issues, although I had minimised this by seeing Ms Green at the office when all the children, except Rose, were at school. I had pointed out to Ms Green something I had observed from many past visits, that when we were discussing matters in the flat, she tended to ignore the approaches of her children, telling them to 'go away, she was talking'. This always made me feel uncomfortable and I felt it gave the children confusing messages; so now instead of merely observing, I would gently suggest that perhaps with the younger ones she could simply hold them or let them sit on her lap, and with the older children, to explain that she was talking to me and she would attend to them soon.

Her responses remained inconsistent in this area, particularly if we talked in the kitchen, which was small, and we were standing up. In the living room, however, she was much better at holding the children, responding to their overtures and talking at the same time. Again, I had observed earlier in the year in my mother and child observation how the mother often held her two-year-old for short periods when the child wanted during other conversation. In Fahlberg's (1994) observation checklist for assessing attachment, there are a number of key areas listed: for example, respond to the child's overtures, provide affective comforting, seem aware of the child's needs. In the less structured visits, therefore, I worked on this area of parenting and I saw an improvement. I tried to do this without undermining her in front of the children. Again, drawing on material from sessions with Asen (1996) on the Goldsmiths course, I used phrases like "notice that Rose is trying to show you something", giving her the cue to pick Rose up. This is a technique I used on a number of visits.

Evaluation of the work

In general, I think that my intervention was successful for a number of reasons. Firstly, for myself, I now feel that I have a much fuller picture of how this family functions and, using principally attachment theory, I can evaluate much better the quality of the children's attachment to their mother. Given the complexity of assessing this, I cannot say that the children fall neatly into categories. However, using Fahlberg's observation checklist, I could identify that while none of the children fulfil all the criteria for secure attachment, there were many elements which indicated good attachment.

My greatest concern, and Ms Green's, at present, is for the eldest child Larry, whom I said earlier was the child least involved in this work. On reflection, one of the difficulties was perhaps that the type of activity did not interest him as a 12-year-old; he said at one session, "Is there anything for me?" I found it difficult to engage him, which surprised me. However, a few weeks later when I returned after my holiday I had a very revealing visit, when I went with the express purpose of seeing

Larry and Helen, the two eldest children. At this stage I was evaluating my work. I spoke to them together and Larry revealed how, since Martin left home, there were no boys around; it was all girls and he had nobody to play with. On top of this, there was considerable sibling rivalry between Helen and Larry, with Helen saying, "Boys are ugly and shout a lot", and Larry accusing Helen of going into his room all the time and messing about with his personal things.

I felt very sad at Helen's comment about her brother Larry. He was extremely upset and the visit ended with Larry being cuddled by his mother. I was wondering whether I had reinforced Larry's sense of isolation within the family by not attempting to engage him more earlier on in the work. In terms of the younger children, I believe there are areas of their development that can be improved, for example with Rose and Kim, their language is delayed and generally there is a need to improve their concentration skills, which I hope will develop if Ms Green is able to continue to develop her own parenting skills.

In general I feel that the situation now is more contained, not only because Martin is absent, but because there is more structure and routine to the children's lives. Also, my direct input into the system and confidence to tackle issues has, I believe, altered the family's functioning to the extent that Ms Green has shown in the sessions a greater ability to interact positively with her children.

For Ms Green, I believe I managed to increase her confidence in her own abilities as a parent. I managed to help her to engage more actively with her children and get down to their level in the play sessions by sitting on the floor with them, which is something I had never seen before. She is paying more attention to the individual needs of the children; in the past she would come to me instantly if she identified a 'problem' with one of them.

Recently, however, in speaking individually to Larry, she discovered he has been glue sniffing; and in talking with Kim she found out she is missing her brother Martin. In July Ms Green learnt she is to move to a new six-bedroom property in the same neighbourhood. While on the one hand she has been feeling overwhelmed by the practical difficulties of furnishing and decorating the property, she has also been giving a lot of thought to planning the space for the children, and involving Larry and Helen in choosing paint colours for their rooms. She has also paid careful attention to safety aspects, given that there are two flights of stairs; and she has designated one room for a playroom, instead of a 'utility' room.

Ms Green, as well as committing herself to the work we have

undertaken in recent months, has also been able to maintain regular contact with Martin, who is still 'accommodated'. She has been visiting a number of schools with me which has meant she has been involved in making the choice for him as well. Together we have identified a placement. Obviously, I have put in a sustained and planned period of work with Ms Green and her children, so I am left wondering what will happen when input is reduced as it inevitably will be in the near future.

As the work has progressed her relationship with her new boyfriend, John, has developed and he appears to be well liked by the children. Ms Green is clearly happier and more confident in this relationship than her last one with Rose's father; this is crucial, I believe, in terms of her ability to manage day-to-day living, while at the same time, attending to the day-to-day needs of her children. For her evaluation of the work see Appendix 1. I asked Ms Green for this contribution. I hope to be in a position to evaluate the work more fully and plan future work after the next case conference is held, which, with good attendance, will give me a more rounded picture of the situation.

What I have learnt

The most valuable experience for me has been the struggle to integrate the theory and practice into my work, using a family where there are so many different dimensions to the work. Although, reflecting back, there are still outstanding issues, I believe that looking at the family as a whole, instead of just its individual parts, has been a tremendous learning experience. Borrowing ideas from the systems approach and using a variety of theoretical/experiential models has given me the confidence to persist with the work, even though at times there have been diversions and interruptions.

The pace of the work has been slower than I would have hoped, mainly due to Martin's absconding, the move to the new house, and children being on holiday. I feel that this is inevitable in working within area fieldwork, where crises and other priorities take precedence over this type of work. Using attachment theory gave me a good base on which to make an assessment of the family functioning, both in terms of the individual children, mother–child relationships, and relations between the children, and enabled me to keep a focus on the children.

On reflection, I should have put more thought into including the eldest child in 'play' sessions, and checked out earlier with the eldest children, Larry and Helen, their feelings now that Martin was no longer at home. Knowing that there had been considerable friction between all three prior to his being accommodated, I falsely assumed that they were probably relieved in the early stages, but perhaps that was a reflection of my own feelings of not constantly being asked to intervene by Ms Green or other professionals 'to sort out Martin'.

When I embarked on the work my knowledge and intuition had told me that Ms Green did have the ability to parent her children with appropriate support and advice. The more systematic approach I adopted confirmed this belief. However, I had the benefit of extensive previous knowledge of the family. I think that when offering services to families we need to explore more fully with them the type of service we are offering, for example psychodynamic, behavioural or task centred, if we are to engage families more successfully. Often when we are involved with families it is not their first contact with social services or other local services, and just as social workers have a preference for adopting a particular approach to the work (in my case task centred) families should also, if possible, be given a preference.

Inevitably, my work with this family will continue and I will have to re-evaluate the family situation and plan future work. Given that Martin is 'accommodated', there will be continuing long-term social work involvement with the family. However, I believe that we have to work towards a situation where the focus of the work is on Martin and his reintegration into the family (we know that he will be starting his new placement in the next two months). At the moment it is difficult to envisage Ms Green being able to manage without much support from social services and having many other professionals involved in the family. Careful consideration has to be given, in the future, as to how a less dependent relationship can be developed.

I am assuming here that all the children's names will be removed from the borough's child protection register in the near future. Continuing with a more systems orientated approach will, I hope, enable us to move towards a situation where Ms Green and her children are able to elicit support from community orientated services and networks. I see this as vital, given her dependency on me and social services at the moment. Also, my understanding is that Ms Green's boyfriend, John, will join the family on his release from prison. If this happens, then it is important I engage with him as well.

Finally, in terms of working with other families, the knowledge, skills and theory I have developed in this work will, I believe, enable me to carry out more skilled assessments in the future, involving families more in that process rather than just carrying out the traditional monitoring role which is a feature of much area-based work. I recognise, however, that, in assessing attachment, while the literature shows that attachment theory applies across cultures, there are differences in terms of attachment styles. In making assessments on attachment, therefore, one has to be sensitive to the race and culture of families.

Appendix 1: Ms Green's evaluation

I have known Patrick Lonergan for about three years. He started off being my ten-year-old son's social worker, but now he helps me and my other five children. My son Martin had very bad behavioural problems which can lead him into being violent and very abusive. Over the last eight or nine months things deteriorated to such an extent that I asked if my son could be accommodated by the social services, which Patrick agreed to as my other children were being affected badly by Martin's behaviour.

All my children have different levels of emotional problems, which Patrick has helped to try and sort out, by arranging for them to see different professional people who can help them. Also because Martin's behaviour has become so bad, I felt strongly that his only chance to change was to go to a therapeutic boarding school, which Patrick agreed with and has since helped me sort out. Also my social worker helped me get a move to a bigger place which now he is trying to help me sort.

We have had a few disagreements in the past, but most of the time we have been willing to try each other's ideas out. Patrick has been coming round to observe how the children play and act with me altogether. One suggestion he made was for all of us to play with some clay, which we all enjoyed, and he took some photos of me and the children all playing together. Patrick also brought round a load of ideas for games and instructions on how to play them, which can include all the different ages of the children.

We still have a long way to go to being a happy family altogether, but now there is some hope that my son Martin will get the help he badly needs and improve his behaviour, and hope that my other children settle down. I still have a lot of work to do with myself and the kids, but Patrick's help should make it easier.

Carol, Anna and Khadia: Work with a three generation black family

Veronique Faure

Purpose of the intervention

Anna (aged 16, Jamaican) has a child, Khadia (age 3). She became pregnant at the age of 12 by her step–brother Roy (also Jamaican), who was 17 at the time (see genogram, Figure 1). Both Anna and Roy were then living with Anna's mother Carol and their two half–sisters, Clare and Ginette. Roy's father had died five years earlier. Anna had become pregnant at the same time as her mother. Roy first admitted and then denied being Khadia's father. He was prosecuted and found guilty of four charges of unlawful sexual intercourse and sentenced to one year's imprisonment.

Carol was initially supportive to Anna. She decided on Roy's prosecution as a result of his denial that he was Khadia's father, which led to family and community feuds, and allegations that "Anna was probably sleeping with lots of boys". The relationship between Anna and Carol, however, deteriorated, leading to Anna and Khadia being accommodated with a friend.

This broke down after a few months and they were accommodated with a foster carer. This broke down after a year, leading to another placement, which recently also broke down. Anna and Khadia returned to live with Carol against their wishes, as social services did not have another placement to offer. The placements were considered to have broken down as a result of Anna falling out with the carers following arguments around Khadia's care, and the carers' feelings that Anna was failing to take responsibility for Khadia.

Figure 1: Genogram

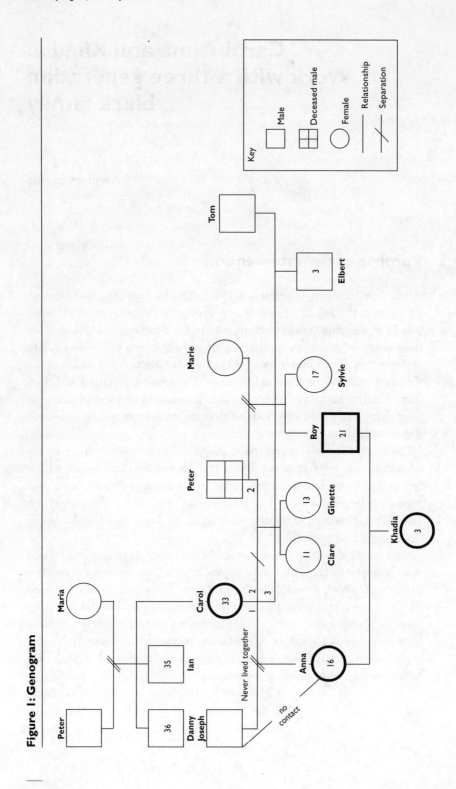

Anna and Khadia's social worker, Maxine (also Jamaican), became concerned that Khadia's needs for stability and consistency were not being met, and about the impact that placement breakdowns were having on her, as well as on Anna (who attends college full time.) Also, a new issue had come to Maxine's attention, in relation to Roy having recently resumed contact with Khadia. Contact was said to take place at the grandmother's house, supervised by Carol and Anna.

Due to pressure of other work, Maxine had had little time to allocate to Anna and Khadia, other than dealing with numerous practical issues and offering Anna support at times of breakdowns. She had been working with them for almost a year. She had tried to do work with Anna earlier around her experience and feelings about Roy and Khadia but without success, as Anna was unwilling to explore these issues. Her work with Carol had been mainly to do with seeking her cooperation in making care plans for Anna and Khadia.

Carol was adamant that she could not continue to look after Anna as they did not get on, but was prepared to look after Khadia as long as Anna was accommodated. Anna was happy with this plan. Maxine was also prepared to support the plan as she felt it met Khadia's needs for stability and consistency and Anna's need for space to finish her studies. In the light of Roy resuming contact with Khadia, however, she felt a child protection assessment needed to be carried out and requested a co-worker to do the assessment with her, as she felt she might fail to be objective in the assessment of risk due to her close relationship with the family.

Assessment

Both Anna and her mother Carol had been offered counselling together and separately at the earlier and later stages of social work involvement, but had declined. Anna and Carol both failed to see Anna and Roy's sexual relationship as child sex abuse (CSA). Both had said that Anna had consented to the sexual relationship which was 'not incestuous' as they were only step siblings. Roy's prosecution had been seen by both as a means to force Roy to take responsibility for his paternity.

Anna had been given the choice by her mother of terminating the pregnancy but decided not to, although her mother had made it clear that even if she offered Anna practical support, the baby would be Anna's responsibility. Anna accepted this. Maxine's assessment was that even if Anna had always taken some responsibility for Khadia's care, as she grew up she had started to resent it. This had lead to confusion of roles between her and her carers and to placement breakdowns.

Maxine gave Anna a lot of credit for pursuing her studies and for her educational achievements, and felt that Anna needed to be relieved of Khadia's care. Anna's emotional bond with Khadia was considered to be often very distant, although she could not be faulted for her physical care. Anna and her mother's relationship was also felt to be distant emotionally. Khadia and her grandmother's relationship was considered to be warm and close.

I felt very strongly that the issues in this case had been so numerous and complex over the years that the family, as well as the social workers involved, had colluded with not addressing the issue of CSA, which had remained unresolved. From file notes, it seemed no groundwork had been done about CSA and I believed this to be causal to Anna/Carol's and Anna/Khadia's poor relationships. Also, if Khadia was to remain in their care, they had to be aware of the risk presented by Roy, not only to Khadia, but also to Anna's sisters who were now much the same age that Anna was at the time of the abuse.

My starting point was that Anna and Roy's sexual relationship was undoubtedly a case of CSA, as Anna, aged 12, could not have consented to sex whatever her feelings for Roy; and that the relationship was incestuous, even if they were step siblings, as they had been brought up as siblings for eight years. I felt the basic groundwork needed to be done with the family before they could challenge their own beliefs about what constituted CSA. This included sharing findings from research by those who worked with perpetrators of CSA.

Theoretical base and methods used

I approached this work from a feminist perspective on CSA. MacLeod and Saraga (1987) describe the feminist premise about CSA as follows:

> Men, in learning to become men, learn they have a right to be sexually and emotionally serviced by women; they learn that their power can ensure that this happens, and that in order to feel like a man, they have to feel powerful. Within the family, women are relatively powerless in relation to men, and children even more so. (p 24)

While the feminist perspective does not preclude factors such as class, culture or race which may compound the problem, CSA is seen primarily as a problem of gender (the majority of abusers are men), and of how society views male sexuality and dominance (the abuse occurs in 'ordinary' families, not just deviant ones). There are other hypotheses which may be compatible with this analysis, including the concept of abuse as "compensation for perceived lack and loss of power" (Finkelhor, 1984, quoted in VACSG, 1990, p 19) or as "an expression of frustration or anger" (Hartman, 1979, quoted in VACSG, 1990, p 19).

From studies on male perpetrators (for example Wyre, 1987) we learn how the emotionally vulnerable child in the family may be engaged in a trusting relationship, 'groomed' by a process of seduction, of entrapment and isolation, resulting in the child feeling confused and possibly believing (s)he consented to, encouraged and is responsible for the abuse.

It seemed essential in our work with this family that both Anna and Carol understood this process, to break the myth of Anna's consent. The power differentials in Anna and Roy's relationship had to be acknowledged, not only in terms of gender but also of age. It is well established that a majority of sex offenders begin their abusive career in adolescence, and this had to be borne in mind while raising Carol and Anna's awareness of the possibility of Roy re-offending and presenting a risk to Khadia and Anna's sisters.

Maxine and I intended to extend the family work to Anna's sisters at a later stage, as their views and understanding seemed essential in preventing any reoccurrence of abuse within this family.

Process of the work

There were two stages to our work. The first involved a great deal of preparation for our intervention. The second was the actual work with the family, which failed as far as family work is concerned, as the relationship and communication between Carol and Anna completely broke down after our third session.

Preparation

Maxine acknowledged having little practice, experience and knowledge of CSA and felt overwhelmed by the complexity of the issues involved in this case. Although I had worked on a number of CSA cases, done a lot of reading and attended a one-year course at the Portman and Tavistock Clinic (Child Sexual Abuse within the Family: An Inter-Agency Approach, 1991-92), I was by no means an expert on CSA and felt equally anxious at the number of issues to be borne in mind, even if I felt more confident in addressing them. Over a few weeks, I collected a number of articles and books which I had found particularly helpful in understanding the dynamics involved in CSA and shared them with Maxine.

I believed it was important that Maxine felt equally empowered in understanding issues of CSA so that she could fully participate in the work. As a white worker I was anxious not to be oppressive in my joint work with a black colleague and a black family. Maxine's sensitivity to the family's experience of alienation from their past encounters with white workers was a real asset to my developing understanding of anti-discriminatory practice.

Intervention

We met on three occasions with Carol and Anna (at Carol's home). Carol quickly engaged in our work but Anna often remained quiet and silent. We started by dealing with the 'here and now', that is, our child protection concerns about Roy's contact with the family and the risk he might present to children. This was initially dismissed by Carol as she accounted for what she believed had happened between Anna and Roy as 'two teenagers exploring their sexuality'. Maxine and I were able to counteract her beliefs by raising the power differentials in age, gender and sexual maturity between Anna and Roy, leading to power imbalance, and how this, we believed, had been abused by Roy.

Anna stated her very strong, although confused, feelings for Roy and felt she did consent to the sexual relationship. We explored this further, until Anna acknowledged that she felt driven to the sexual relationship and was actually never asked by Roy if this was alright with her. She became very tearful at this point and agreed that if she was not asked, she could not consent.

We worked with Carol's initial stated anger at Roy for what she saw as abuse of *her* trust (she had left him in charge at home while she attended an evening course, which is when the abuse took place). It became clear that Roy had assumed a parental/paternal role in the family as he grew up after his father's death.

As the work carried on we encouraged Anna to become aware also of her anger towards Roy, which she had suppressed because of her guilt about his prison sentence and current inability to find a job because of this. Quite unexpectedly Carol started disclosing issues that were unknown to Maxine and previous social workers: her own history of sexual abuse by her father at the age of 10, the matrimonial violence suffered by her mother who escaped to America a few months after

Carol's disclosure of abuse, and her care history as a result (Anna had knowledge of all of this).

Carol talked about how she had learnt to become detached and unemotional and acknowledged the impact this had had on her relationship with Anna. Anna in turn acknowledged the same process and impact on her relationship with Khadia. Carol's suppressed feelings of guilt became evident to Maxine and me as she talked about how determined she had been to ensure that her children would never go through the same experience of CSA, leading to her rationalisation that Anna and Roy's sexual relationship had nothing to do with CSA.

The day before our fourth session, Anna presented herself as homeless at the office. Her mother had 'chucked her out' after an argument about Anna coming home very late. Khadia was with her, despite Carol offering to keep her. They were accommodated in a hotel with social work support as no other placement was available.

The work currently being done with Anna and Carol, separately as they are not now talking, is around stabilising Khadia's situation, although Anna is now certain that she wants to continue looking after Khadia herself. There is uncertainty still as to whether the family work could be resumed at a later stage.

Evaluation of the intervention

We aimed to work in a way which confronted the family's denial and minimisation of CSA while not being inappropriately oppressive to either Carol or Anna, and in a way which we hoped would validate their feelings of confusion, anger and guilt. Although I believed we partly succeeded in raising their awareness as to what truly happened in their family, denial and minimisation had served a purpose. There had been 'coping/defence mechanisms' which had allowed the family to survive and continue to function, at least in their ability to offer each other practical support.

I feel, however, that Maxine and I failed to evaluate the seriousness, in terms of impact and implications, that shaking a family's belief system would have on the dynamics of individual relationships (not just Carol and Anna's, but also theirs in relation to Khadia, Roy, the extended family and the community). I also question the timing of our intervention. This work needed to have been done earlier, not at a time of crisis when both Anna and Khadia's situations were unsettled. This met the agency's need to carry out a risk assessment at that particular time, which was probably not a safe time for the family, and I fear that it might have further damaged Carol and Anna's relationship.

In Maxine's continued work with Anna, however, what she feels we might have achieved is to have empowered and enabled Anna to feel strong enough to think about confronting her mother and Roy, and stand more independently and confidently in the assessment and decisions she is making about what has happened and what should happen next.

Anna, for instance, has decided that she wants to carry on addressing some of the issues we raised and is seeking counselling. She says she does not want to avoid confronting the issues any more as she wants to be prepared for dealing with Khadia who, as she grows up, will ask questions and need explanations about her parentage.

The work is not concluded. There is no final resolution of any of the issues that still need addressing (in terms of child protection and Khadia's need for consistent parenting and stability), and this is ongoing. What I feel emerged from our work, as practitioners and not as experts, is a true reflection of our striving to come to grips with the various perspectives, theories and skills which we judged to be helpful in working with this family, and effective in enabling them to confront some of their difficulties.

Commentary from an academic perspective

Jane Dutton

Introduction

The lens through which we look at practice can never be value free, and neither can the lens through which these commentaries are made. My own position as a social work lecturer and a family therapist, and my extensive previous professional experience as a social work practitioner and manager in work with children and families, particularly in child protection, and the values and beliefs inherent in this work, must inevitably influence my commentary.

The opportunity for experienced practitioners to reflect, learn and creatively develop their practice is essential to the development of high quality services. This opportunity is clearly in evidence in these accounts.

Mary Cody
The Phillips family: An adoption assessment

The writing style of the assessment is engaging, explicit and interesting. Indeed, the style itself could be seen to reflect the open transaction with the family which the author is aiming for. The work is centrally concerned with developing a partnership approach. Negotiating this indicates the author's understanding of the power dynamics, balances and imbalances, which inevitably underpin the work throughout. Positioning this discussion at the beginning of the account emphasises its importance. It would have been useful to have some specific examples or brief excerpts of dialogue at this point, to illustrate the family's understanding of the power they individually and collectively had, did not have, or sought to develop.

The choice of theoretical perspectives to underpin practice is clearly articulated. Some of these approaches could have been linked. For example, the 1990s have yielded a developing literature on the implications of attachment theory for family systems (Hinde, 1990; Byng-Hall and Hinde, 1991; Donley, 1993). Byng-Hall (1995) defines a secure family base as:

> ... a family that provides a reliable network of attachment relationships which enables all family members of whatever age to feel sufficiently secure to explore relationships with each other and with others outside the family. (p 19)

Developing a further theoretical coherence in this way could contribute to the author's work in developing with the family coherent and accessible stories about their experiences of the adoption process.

The practice described in the two sessions, in considering how the adoptive parents might help the child understand and integrate his or her own previous life story into current experience is, in my view, the fundamental strength of this piece of work. Using the ecomap and genogram as tools to make visible the complicated concerns about the balance between stress and support, individual and collective needs, loss and grief and significant attachments enabled the whole family to talk about and listen to powerful feelings. The author demonstrated an ability to facilitate the family's explanation, rather than provide or assume interpretations of her own.

Additionally, she was able to reflect on her own position in this work system. She raises a crucial dilemma in identifying her concern about the implications of her task setting with the adoptive parents. The aim was to facilitate their thinking further about some of the complexities of birth parents' lives and how these may have affected their behaviour. For the practitioner, mindful of the best interests of the child to be placed, there may be an understandably powerful wish for the adoptive parents to show sympathy for birth parents, particularly as research would indicate that this has positive effects on placement outcome.

The conflict and ambivalence that adoptive parents may feel, however, is also understandable. One possible way forward with this dilemma may have been to return to theoretical perspectives. Systems thinking particularly emphasises the impact of the worker's own value system on the work. It also introduces the possibility of multiple positions. Using this perspective to reflect on how the practitioner's concern, however valid, may be organising the work or going too fast, potentially creates space for the adoptive parents' ambivalence and confusion to be acknowledged as real and important to them.

It also allows the possibility of differences between them to be validated, inhibiting the potential for one parent being assessed more favourably than the other. As the author reflects, unravelling the meaning of these feelings and how they might impact on family life creates a greater possibility of moving on over time, and of helping the child with their inevitable ambivalences and confusions.

These reflections demonstrate a lively sensitivity to the work. Strengthening the relationship between theory and practice, would have added to this rich and rewarding account.

Stephen Kitchman
The Drays: Breaking the pattern of reactive behaviour

This is an important practice example, highlighting as it does the key tensions in social work with children and families in the current social, political, economic and organisational climate. The family's 'chaos' threatens to 'swamp' the worker and the agency. The children and each parent have powerful individual needs, and the family as a unit has practical, financial and emotional needs. The balance between family support and child protection is uneasily held (Parton, 1997).

Other professionals' unspecified fears and the pattern of incidents concerning three of the children indicate serious protection concerns (DoH, 1991a). Within the agency, there is a will to initially work preventatively to try to alleviate pressure and explore the potential for increased protection (1989 Children Act, Part III).

The author has worked hard to order the material into a coherent account. The struggle to establish coherence in practice is reflected in the writing. As the allocated worker, it is often difficult to create sufficient distance from the chaos to be able to observe patterns of behaviour. Theoretical perspectives are essential tools in facilitating this process of developing sufficient clarity to practice effectively in a chaotic context. Several perspectives are referred to in the text and it would have been worth expanding on these in order to further illustrate the complicated balance which is inherently part of such work.

The significance of the relationship between the family and social services may be understood from different perspectives (Mattinson and Sinclair, 1979; Dale, 1988), but the notion of social services as parent is clearly important. Both parents here carry a history of social services as their carers and have a present reality of the agency in the parental role of providing support. The position of the worker as the potential representative of parental authority, therefore, becomes central. The parents' possible ambivalence and struggle with this representation will also maintain them in a particular position, making it difficult for them to move on in spite of the worker's best efforts and their own expressed wish to do so (for a further analysis, see Burnham, 1986).

The author also comments on the importance of attachment in this situation. He particularly refers to concern about attachment between the children and their parents. The research he uses (Mattinson and Sinclair, 1979) also comments on the anxious and ambivalent attachment which often exists between couples in such positions. Threats of separation and violence are frequent:

> Anger and anxiety, need and aggression follow on each other's heels
> in ways calculated to confuse and exasperate the outsider. Crises
> characterise the lives of such families. (Howe, 1995, p 156)

In such contexts, there is a strong need for each parent to ally with the social worker to draw them into the couple relationship, as demonstrated in this situation.

The practice dilemmas examined in the text highlighted the need for the worker to be aware of gender and power imbalances, to reinforce the importance of the parents working together and avoid collusion with either, while maintaining a child-focused approach. The impact on the worker of holding these balances is alluded to, and could be analysed further, particularly as this also in turn impacts on the work as part of a reflexive process (Burnham, 1986).

Supervision is crucial, as acknowledged here and reported elsewhere (Blom Cooper, 1985). The supervisory relationship itself, however, may mirror the relationship between worker and family, and is a crucial consideration in developing a reflective practice.

This piece of work has finely illustrated the complexity of understanding and working with the delicate balance of need, support, prevention and protection, which is the everyday experience of social work with children and families.

Michael Atkinson
The Reids: Putting boundaries in place

The author has established a coherent theoretical framework within which he can examine with the family their boundary setting, experiences of dyadic and triadic relationships, and sense of personal safety. His organisation of the material gives a clear and detailed study of his practice with the family. Incorporating examples of his own questions and different family members' comments and responses invites the reader's involvement in a dynamic and engaging way.

One of the key themes to emerge is that of generational patterns in relation to gender and power. Male violence towards women and children, and damaged attachments between parent and child, emerge as patterns for each parent. Both had difficult and disempowering family experiences as children. The author considers these patterns theoretically and in practice. Their centrality in this work, however, would suggest further analysis of the individual belief systems that the couple brought with them into this relationship, and the way these may have constructed beliefs and action in relation to power and powerlessness in the current family context. The different levels of equality held by family members in relation to the degree of choice they may have about adhering to or influencing the ground rules of the family group (Barnes, 1995) is a thread running through the work, and a more detailed theoretical analysis would do greater justice to the practice.

The gender and value systems of the worker are particularly relevant in such work. The author acknowledges his awareness of the potential bids for an alliance with him from each of the couple, and indicates where the power of the system unbalanced his 'neutrality'. The way in which his male professional power is understood by other professionals and family members forms part of his analysis of power relations in the system, and how these dynamics influence outcomes.

The process of the work amply demonstrated the author's use of systemic thinking and techniques. His use of questioning encouraged the father into taking a more parental position, and the enactment demonstrated the power and the inconsistency of the couple coalition and its effect on their son. Working on the relationship between internal and external worlds with all three, and making this visible to each, demonstrated the boy's emotional vulnerability and encouraged responses from the adults.

They, in turn, had further space as a couple to explore generational patterns they experienced as destructive. It may have been useful here to develop this work further, moving from understanding the impact of these patterns on their current relationship and family life to starting to 'rewrite family scripts' (Byng-Hall, 1995).

A strength in this work is the author's openness to considering individual family member's needs. These were addressed within the family work, but in evaluating this the author also acknowledges the extent of individual needs and looks at addressing ways to resource these. This is a different way of connecting internal and external worlds or realities and an appropriate use of professional authority.

The learning points ably summarise the key themes of the work. A particularly important reflection is on the potential for the abuse of power by the worker. Understanding this in practice, and taking action immediately, addressed the central theme of safety and offered a model of self-control in this volatile situation.

Patrick Lonergan
The Green family: Work with a lone parent and her children

One of the values of this piece of work is the way in which it demonstrates introducing a different approach in the context of a long-term piece of work. Over time, a worker may accommodate to aspects of family life, miss new information or accept little change. The worker may assume something of the role of the absent parent in working with a lone-parent family. In this scenario, both worker and parent may have felt 'defeated' by her son's behaviour and by the demands of the large family. With the worker undertaking further professional training, however, there was the possibility of returning to the work with a 'fresh pair of eyes'.

A consistent theme in this engaging piece of writing is the author's affirmation of the parent's commitment to her children, ability to sustain that commitment and to work with professionals on their behalf. That affirmation must influence the relationship and contribute to developing trust. Although all the children's names were in the child protection register, the author has chosen to identify them as 'children in need' (Children Act 1989, Section 17), and work with the family within this framework, notwithstanding one son's accommodation (Children Act 1989, Section 20). This decision must also affect the climate for working together.

The choice of theoretical perspectives took account of previous work and the family's responses to it. Systemic thinking and attachment theory both seem highly relevant here. These perspectives could have been discussed further to include, for example, ideas on a parent's own attachments over time in the context of childhood and previous couple relationships (Mattinson and Sinclair, 1979; Byng-Hall, 1995). The genogram work could also perhaps have been developed, using systemic thinking to explore, for example, what was happening for individual family members around the time of each birth.

The sensitivity of the author to the importance of his position in this work was crucial. He acknowledges this in his section on anti-discriminatory practice and in his evaluation. Both his gender and his role imbued him with a considerable amount of power, which notions of working in partnership and empowering practice cannot alter. Understanding the ways in which the role, and in this case gender, may affect the work, however, can critically influence this power imbalance if there is open discussion with the client (Burck and Speed, 1995).

Observation and direct work with the family demonstrated a useful combination of theoretical frameworks informing the practice, which in turn was practical, specific, accessible and applicable. The issue of dependency and independence often creates a tension for workers. The author deals with this by maintaining a balance between using the client's own insight and strengths, making suggestions or asking questions, and offering practical assistance. Setting joint achievable goals within the financial and emotional constraints of the situation allowed the client to take further control, but at the same time feel supported and validated for the real efforts she was making.

Maintaining a sharper systemic edge to the work might have brought the eldest boy's sense of isolation, and the impact of his brother's leaving, more sharply into the frame of work. Loss, particularly the loss of males, is a recurrent theme in this family and spending time discussing this with them might facilitate the transitions they are, and will be, facing. Thinking about loss and change is sometimes challenging for the worker, who may be keenly aware of their own position in the family system and how the family might experience their departure when the work ends.

Using his own response to the initial chaos he experienced in observing the family together led the author to consider how they might feel about it. Reflecting on his own shift in response as some routine was introduced seemed congruent with his observation of the family appearing more contained. Monitoring personal responses to the work is an important component of reflective practice, and may challenge potential assumptions based on racial, cultural, class or other differences or similarities between worker and family.

Veronique Faure
Carol, Anna and Khadia: Work with a three generation black family

This piece of work is written with a clarity which is often hard to achieve when discussing the complexity of child sexual abuse. Relationships between the professional system and the family, and between the family members, are frequently confused, with boundaries inappropriately drawn. The author has given an honest account of these relationships. The work itself highlights a consistently important issue in statutory work with children and families. It is into this context that the family is referred, often in a raw state, and it is often at this point that important therapeutically orientated work could be done. Organisationally this is often not possible, as in this case, with ensuing complications and often further damage.

Changes in the professional system or decision making often reflect shifts in the family system. In this instance, a re-emergence of protection concerns meant that co-work was requested and agreed. Starting this relationship is in itself complicated, as the author indicates. Exploring the complexity further might have been useful in developing thinking together about the possible impact of intervention. In a practice situation where power issues are paramount, these will inevitably be reflected in the co-work pair. The racial and cultural difference between the workers, their different relationship to the family and different levels of experience in working with child sexual abuse, all create the potential for mistrust and misunderstanding between them (Burnham and Harris, 1997).

The preparation for such work then will need to be carefully allowed for. The author gives an indication of this here, but it would have been useful to have a more detailed analysis of the necessary thinking about differences and similarities between the workers, strengths they each might bring to the situation and the possible pitfalls. These might include a potential for inappropriate alliances, splitting into 'good' and 'bad' workers, boundary confusion, feeling silenced or isolated, powerless and marginalised. The vulnerability of the professional system to reflecting the dynamics of the family system in such situations may be acutely experienced in the co-work relationship. Preparation and time to discuss sessions afterwards are, therefore, essential, but may not be allowed for by the organisation, leaving both workers feeling abused and powerless. A further level of reflective analysis on these processes would have done more justice to the practice.

The crucial decision here in creating a difference was to focus and maintain that focus on the abuse as abuse, and not as consensual sex. The grandmother's emerging story was then able to give new meaning to closeness and intimacy as potentially dangerous. Maintaining emotional distance as a way of managing this danger seemed to be a pattern repeating over time (Jones, 1991). It might, therefore, have been useful in the sessions to name and explore the possibility of having to separate if mother and daughter became too close.

Drawing out repeating generational patterns and thinking about how to use this information in practice implies time to reflect and access to supervision or consultation. It was not clear whether the workers had access to this. Without it, it is difficult to maintain sufficient distance from the work and manage the feelings engendered by it, to observe and reflect on new information and emerging patterns.

The author's evaluation thoughtfully addressed some of these issues. She also commented on the fact that the work was not concluded: there were no final resolutions to record. This is an important point to have made. Social workers are more often involved in complex processes than in neat final resolutions, and this was a good example of working positively with uncertainty and ambiguity.

Reflecting on the commentaries

Each of these pieces of work demonstrates a vibrant enjoyment of learning and applying this learning creatively to practice. They address the gap between the "high ground" of academic rigour and "the swampy lowlands of practice" (Schon, 1987, p 3). Each text emphasises the importance of working in partnership as an example of good practice, as well as following the current tenets of law and policy. There is a partnership in learning demonstrated here also.

Transitional points in the life cycle of individuals and families are vividly described in the writing. For the practitioners themselves, managing the inevitable process of change which comes through learning and the opportunity for reflection is a powerful subtext. Continuity and discontinuity are addressed in each piece of work, and are also part of the learning process. The emphasis on reflection has provided the opportunity to hold and contain these processes and maximise capacities for critical thinking.

A focus for each piece of work was the relationship around the presenting difficulty. These commentaries also focused on relationship: the relationship between the issue, family, agency, theory and practice, and reflection on the work. The complexity of each situation was such, however, that each commentary only related to a small corner of a much larger canvas.

The theoretical concepts most frequently used were attachment theory and systemic thinking. Planning interventions with complex family and professional systems, and considering the impact of generational patterns of attachment on current difficulties, made these appropriate choices in this area of work. Interestingly, none of the authors used texts which link some of this thinking (Byng-Hall, 1995; Barnes, 1995). Choosing these frameworks to facilitate practice which is so clearly grounded in the reality of social work with children and families today highlights the importance of centrally addressing these theories in social work training.

One of the most consistent themes in the practice was the complexity of working with violence. Physical abuse, sexual abuse, emotional abuse and the impact of domestic violence were present in all but one of the texts. In that one the impact of loss and trauma on the adoptive child and family was an essential element of the work. This significantly demonstrates the complex and often distressing and anxiety provoking nature of ordinary work with children and their families. In the social work context, the extraordinary may become ordinary. For a large proportion of the population these are media stories. For social workers and those with whom they work, these are their personal and professional lives.

Commentary from a practitioner perspective

Sigurd Reimers

Within the family therapy field these days one tends to talk more about systemic thinking and less about systems theory. This could be an important shift for those social workers who are interested in developing a more systemic practice. Systems theory originated in the physical sciences, and claimed that systems could be measured accurately, and that the parts of any system behaved in a predictable, and rather mechanistic way. At that time (1950s to 1970s) this was a useful development in that it helped us think of how the behaviour of one part of a system (like the family) influenced that of others, and allowed us to move away from over-focusing on the isolated individual.

However, by the end of the 1970s it was becoming clearer that what might work in physics with inanimate objects might not apply so neatly to the complex situations facing human beings (Hoffman, 1990). Systemic thinking, by contrast, has come to emphasise how the thoughts, beliefs and meanings held by individuals and shared by important others within a system may form a pattern, but are often quite unpredictable, especially within complex systems such as many of the families with whom social workers are working.

This puts us less in the position of being experts, and more of being explorers. We may even become co-explorers with our clients, if we play our cards right and our clients and agencies permit.

The consequences of this shift in thinking can be immense. How can we, as agents of the state, any longer be as confident as we used to be in assessing people and difficult situations, if we are no longer expert outside observers? This was a dilemma faced in most of the case examples described. Although the authors were careful not to claim expert powers, they were grappling with the fact that we are all often required to act as if we are experts at how people should conduct their lives, and we therefore run the risk of overstepping the mark. Systemic thinking suggests that we take the trouble from time to time to challenge anything that passes for expertise, especially when this ends up being simplistic and dogmatic.

An idea which can help us not oversimplify complicated situations is that of the double description (Bateson, 1972). This encourages us to consider carefully two or more accounts of the same situation. The dominant account (sometimes called a 'narrative' or 'story') (White and Epston, 1990) may be one of abuse, violence, and crime – issues which the state often requires its social workers to handle. A different type of account (sometimes called 'subjugated') may be one to do with generations of oppression within families, or of oppression towards families by the state itself.

Subjugated stories are often not expressed or have got lost. They are frequently tragic and finely detailed, and may need talking about and being listened to. In this process the strengths within individuals and families become acknowledged and some modest hope is offered. A respectful focusing on strengths is in itself a good context for promoting change, while blame and directiveness are often ineffective.

But which is the correct or the best story? Systemic thinkers would say that we cannot know with certainty, but that if empowerment is to mean anything, it must mean creating a thinking and a talking space within which these 'lost' stories can be developed. Also, because the stories of any individual connect with those of other individuals, the family can be a good setting within which to share, and even disagree, about these stories. This process may encourage people to adjust some of their more destructive stories and start living a new and more hopeful one.

To achieve a viable double description, social workers (and other agents of the state) may have to strike a careful balance. On the one hand, stories of abuse, madness and crime (public stories) may need to be acted on if particularly vulnerable individuals within the family (whose stories are perhaps the most subjugated of all) are to be protected. We have the law, agency policies and procedures to remind us of this. On the other hand, clients who are needing to be controlled in some way may also benefit from an opportunity to develop and control their own private stories. Without this second part of the process, we are likely to become oppressive as we increasingly impose our views and agendas, rather than encourage people to develop theirs (Howe, 1987).

What we see at times in the case examples presented here are attempts to allow such a space for thinking, talking and listening to develop. These attempts are mostly set within a context of chaos, hopelessness and public resignation, which are factors that can prevent the process of change.

In these accounts we see how much social work draws on attachment theory. This theory encourages us to be attentive to the early life experiences of clients, and how these can make a difference to how attachments are developed in the next generation. Attachment theory, which has not developed within the systemic field, can be useful to social workers because it offers some ideas about what may be some of the limitations we can expect from clients as parents of dependent children.

We should, however, be careful about assuming that it is inevitable that the next generation will turn out like the previous one, merely because of poor attachment in childhood (Rutter, 1999). A belief in history can provide a degree of realism, but it can also become oppressive. If we become too attached to such beliefs, we may stop believing that change can take place, and that will become evident in our attitudes to our clients.

Everything has to be understood as happening within a context, and that includes family work itself. Any worker trying anything new or unusual (which may include family work) needs to check carefully where such a venture might fit within his/her agency and the wider welfare field. It is important to look over our shoulders! Systemic thinking involves examining our professional and management systems (not forgetting ourselves) as carefully as those of the families we encounter. The term 'dysfunctional family' has its limitations because it oversimplifies, treats families as if they were physical objects and ignores their competence. It also allows us to forget about the part played by our own 'dysfunctions' (stereotypes and other forms of state abuse of power) and those of our agencies.

In working with families we usually focus on the here and now in some detail. But we also have to consider the historical perspective (another double description), and not least what beliefs (Dallos, 1991) people operating within the problem system (including ourselves again) currently hold about their history.

Because members in any system influence each other, it is important that we are open to feedback to our actions from our clients, our agency and other agencies. This feedback may influence what kind of interviewing format we decide to use. We may prefer to work with the whole family (although these days the term 'family' can be hard to define conclusively), and this may prove helpful. However, feedback may suggest that we should use other formats as well, for instance meeting couples, other parts of the family, or individuals. If we feel we are failing with using a particular format (and incidentally family members may be feeling the same), we may use this feedback to consider a different format. This may help a stuck system develop new and more hopeful stories. And in the end we all live our lives according to our stories.

Mary Cody
The Phillips family: An adoption assessment

In this example we see the importance of acknowledging the power of the worker when making assessments. This power calls for sensitivity and clear thinking on the part of the worker if 'partnership' and sharing are not to become slogans designed to reassure the worker. This acknowledgement has two parts – firstly to be clear in one's own mind about one's role, and secondly to express this clearly to one's clients.

There are times when we need to be explicit with our clients about the presence of inbuilt conflicts of interest within the adoption system – between the adult applicants who desperately want a child, and the state (social worker) which is required to assess the suitability of (and sometimes reject) adoption applicants. Without such a clear acknowledgement applicants, who are in a less powerful position within the system, are more likely to resort to controlling the supply of adverse information (the one area in which they are powerful) without which the assessment cannot be accurate. Withholding or distorting information is always an option, and so is being open and making oneself vulnerable to the state. The choice may not always be easy for the best of us, and social workers who feel cornered by deceitful clients do well to consider the logic behind such behaviour.

We see a good example here of a worker trying not to impose an idea of a normative family (what good adoptive families should be like). We can, however, and perhaps should, never be totally neutral, but we can try to become more aware of our norms and therefore use these norms with less prejudice. There were references to the worker's (and perhaps the agency's) norms about what are desirable personal attributes and family processes, for instance the importance of adoptive parents understanding their own ambivalent feelings about adopted children's birth parents, a value and respect for children, and an acknowledgement of their own losses.

In this case the worker and the family were able to form a good working relationship, but what about those cases where such a relationship does not develop, or when the desirable attributes and processes are not present? In such situations the worker's system faces the dilemma of whether to reject the application (on the basis of its values and ideas about what is good for adoptive children), or to revise some of its existing ideas and values. After all, no values remain absolute in all their details for ever.

We also see some techniques which could help with the assessment process (Manor, 1984). The genogram (family tree) is described as a powerful and emotive tool. It should, therefore, never be used in a standard administrative fashion. It is a very personal form of self-exposure, and in this case we heard a sad story of, among other things, dead children and other losses. Any adoption worker might find it hard not to impose a simple interpretation on such details. It may be better to tolerate a dilemma based on the tension between one's own expert ideas (informed by research and our own experience), and being curious about the applicant's own beliefs about important family events.

There was also a reference to the use of enactment. This powerful technique can be a good way of encouraging the worker not to be too central and letting families take responsibility for their own conversation by talking directly to each other in the presence of the worker. An enactment can play a part in helping us assess relationships. But it can also lead to vulnerable people feeling blamed and stereotyped. Such a use of power on the part of the worker (Treacher and Carpenter, 1993) may need to be tempered with allowing their own account to be developed in conversation with the worker.

Stephen Kitchman
The Drays: Breaking the pattern of reactive behaviour

Social workers often aim to see family members together. In this example the aim of family work was to gain an insight into what the household was normally like and to put the children more at their ease. Family interviews can serve a double function. Firstly the worker can check his own perceptions against the accounts of individual members. This may be essential if one has a statutory responsibility for setting certain minimum standards of childcare (Reder et al, 1993), or to assess the need for support services.

However, such assessments have to be balanced against the fact that our very presence cannot help changing the way people usually relate to each other, and also that we will to some extent always bring our own favourite ideas about what we are observing. These are both tendencies which we need to check carefully, and the reference to subjectivity in the account is an important recognition of this.

The second function of a family interview is to be a powerful intervention in its own right. After all, it is rare for any agency of the state to be invited to meet a whole family, and many families never sit down, even with each other, to talk together about their concerns. The initial message from the worker thinking of starting to do family work should be one of an official and positive recognition of them as a family unit. This may go some way, especially within the context of statutory responsibilities, to counter their perception of themselves as a unit of failure (Carpenter, 1996).

When working systemically, we all have to consider our own attitudes to change. Who is responsible for change, the worker or the family? In this example we hear of social services almost becoming like a parent, as if they could single-handedly bring about change. The actual parents started by imposing their different agendas (the mother wanted support services and the father wanted his wife and son to change, but without any responsibility on his part).

Either of these agendas might have been viable, and each parent seemed to need an opportunity to speak to the worker on their own. A worker meeting people individually will, however, need to check very carefully what confidences or 'secrets' he is being encouraged to look after in such sessions. He may also need to encourage joint meetings in order to overcome the pressures of acting like a parent himself, unless he has an official mandate (like a court order) for doing so.

An interesting question of gender was raised. This can be viewed as one important form of structured difference and power. I believe that it is generally good for male workers (and female workers) to try and engage with men in families (as well as with women). Men often feel marginal within their families (Kramer, 1995), and their silence can be extremely powerful. But their silence can also result from feeling total outsiders. Engaging men in family work is often crucial to promoting change, because it gives them recognition at the same time as stressing male responsibility.

We may need to be attentive to the contributions of both genders, but there can also be exceptions to this, as to any rule. For instance, in family work some men become overbearing and remain stubbornly dominant, and women may feel undermined in the one area (talking) where they have previously felt competent. What is best to do in such a situation depends on our attentiveness to feedback to our attempts to bring people together to talk.

Michael Atkinson
The Reids: Putting boundaries in place

This account illustrates some of the difficulties faced when colleagues hold very different opinions from each other. One of the advantages of focusing on wider systems than the family is that any professional within the problem system – or the so-called 'problem-organised system' (Anderson and Goolishian, 1988) – can be as much part of the problem as the family is. That must include colleagues, agencies and even ourselves (Reimers and Street, 1993). An accurate assessment of the nature of this system is particularly important where there are many agencies involved, but also, as is clearly implied here, where the history of 'help' has been a long and controversial one. We sometimes ignore history at our peril.

How do we encourage people (especially men) to talk about matters that may be troubling them, especially when we are led to believe that such talking can sometimes provide relief? Perhaps we have to recognise that no intervention works equally well in all situations. Actively recognising a client's privacy, say around his/her own experiences of childhood abuse, can be a liberating experience, especially if accompanied by a clear hint that the worker would respect the client if he/she later decided to talk.

Addressing gender issues (or other issues relating to structured power) can give workers an opportunity to help people develop more appropriate boundaries. This may in turn promote change. In this case it could be important to draw a boundary between men taking sole responsibility for their violent behaviour on the one hand, and the joint responsibility between both partners for parenting and their relationship on the other (Goldner et al, 1990). Schedule 1 status is intended to warn us of specific dangers to children, not to demonise the individual. This may be easier said than done, since the rest of the problem system may – out of fear of collusion – be pushing the worker to blame the client in a global fashion. It is interesting to see how the worker and the family in this case were able to move away from such a stance.

When we consider doing 'family work' we are immediately confronted with the question of how widely we should define the 'family' (Muncie and Sapsford, 1993), and even how desirable it is. Some family relationships work best when family members live in different households. This is why the term 'transformation' is sometimes preferable to 'family breakdown'. In the end family work may be more about finding an interview format (or a shifting combination of formats) which focuses more on the quality of relationships than on household composition.

This may require all the participants within a diffuse system to become clearer with each other about their roles in relation to each other. Children are often confused because no one has spoken clearly to them. Individual work may also play a helpful part in this process, providing the worker communicates adequately with others in the system and does not come to be seen as a competing parent.

Patrick Lonergan
The Green family: Work with a lone parent and her children

Joint work is raised as an important issue, and this is one which is taken seriously in systemic practice. It is a sad irony that social work is the very setting which might seem to benefit the most from this, but has little tradition of joint work and few opportunities for practising it. Joint work is about mutual support for workers, but is also an opportunity to introduce 'difference' (new thoughts and ideas) as a way of promoting change. A powerful problem-saturated story is easier to challenge if one is not exclusively working (and thinking) single-handedly. New and more hopeful ideas and stories can often emerge when one is working with someone else, possibly of a different gender, generation or race, or one who simply takes more of a back seat role and shares his/her views at the end of an interview.

In order to capitalise most on this sense of difference, the observer may sit a little on the outside of the interviewing circle and offer a different angle on the stuck situation which is being talked about (Smith and Kingston, 1980). Any joint work requires the workers to examine their respective roles carefully so that they do not end up accidentally mirroring conflicts within the family, or family members mirroring those of the workers.

We have already seen that action techniques can play a useful part in family work, but there is also a case for periods of quiet reflection (Burnham, 1986), particularly in those situations (often on home visits!) where people use action – any action – to avoid reflecting on their anxieties and miseries. Where a particular interview format becomes unmanageable (for example, endless chaotic family sessions or defensive individual sessions), this fact may act as useful feedback to the worker and suggest that a different, and more reflective, format be considered.

Many social workers have the double role of carrying out family work as a problem-solving exercise as well as assessing for child protection purposes or for the provision of services, like accommodation for children. They have to pay careful attention to the dilemmas that this may entail (Dungworth and Reimers, 1984). Clients within a problem system often face a corresponding dilemma of whether to face the discomfort of working at change within their family relationships or seeking a solution (sometimes a distraction) through the use of services. In practice, either solution may be valid.

As an example of support services, accommodation may be one way of creating a more adequate distance within a situation that has become too intense. But, in addition, family work may be a way of developing and monitoring a more appropriate distance, which will allow for family members to find the best combination of connectedness and independence. In doing this the worker may need to try and adopt a fairly neutral stance (that is, one that is not too certain about what should be the desired outcome). Certainty can be an attractive option for people working in chaotic circumstances, particularly when one is relating to people who have come to overdepend on the state as a parent (Jordan, 1979), but often fails in highly complex situations.

Veronique Faure
Carol, Anna and Khadia: Work with a three generation black family

This account raises the dilemma of what to do when there is a clash of values between worker and clients (Treacher, 1995). Is 'sexual abuse' equally disastrous for all children? What is the difference between 'sexual abuse' (workers' view) and 'two teenagers exploring their sexuality' (grandmother's and mother's apparent view)? In openly disagreeing with a client who holds a strong view, as we see here, any worker risks alienating her client. Also, the claim to know better (perhaps coming across as too much of an expert or a better parent than the parent) can be oppressive (Corrigan and Leonard, 1978). Yet there are times when a worker will need to take the risk of challenging her client's views, especially when she is working as a representative of the state (and its values) (Dimmock and Dungworth, 1983).

Taking that risk may have been important here. It certainly appears that the experience of being confronted with the beliefs of the two workers may have led the grandmother to talk for the first time about her own childhood experience of sexual abuse. This kind of talking can be very helpful, but it is not automatically good or bad – talking never is. It can connect people or push them apart. Perhaps in this case it played a part in the mother being thrown out of the grandmother's house.

But beyond the crisis of the moment that may possibly not have been such a bad thing. It might have been a way of helping the mother learn self-reliance and of creating a more realistic distance within the family relationship. Many factors will decide that, and workers in such situations need to consider the relative merits of talking and privacy, closeness and distance.

We are told that the family work failed, and two people became homeless in the process. But we cannot expect that family work should always result in people living together more happily. What it can achieve is to provide workers and clients with feedback in their assessment about what is likely to work best at the moment, and that may sometimes be a period of separation.

The question of timing is raised. 'Assessment' (both of what may need to change and what it may be possible to change) and 'family work' (work with families to promote change) sometimes need to be distinct activities. This is particularly so where the state may decide, on the basis of the assessment, to take unpopular action, which makes family work impossible, at least for the time being. In some of those instances it may be better to work for a period with individuals, or with small parts (subsystems) of the family.

We need to remember that everything in professional 'helping' (including our favourite ideas) is provisional – the future in this case may suggest further three-generational sessions along the lines attempted, but at a later stage.

Joint work is an important feature of this case, and the question of racial diversity is raised. Perhaps we should draw a distinction between difference, conflict and oppression. The first may be useful in promoting change, the second may provide energy for that change, but the third will ultimately be self-defeating. Cultural differences can provide pitfalls (as around how to define child abuse), but they can sometimes provide clarity and offer opportunities for oppression to be addressed and for a greater variety of ideas to be applied to stuck situations.

Learning points

Helen Martyn

- Theoretical knowledge and clarity is essential, but theory needs to be applied intelligently, sensitively and flexibility.
- Skilled and appropriate supervision is crucial, as is time for a reflective discussion between workers.
- The power of the worker should always be recognised and acknowledged, as should the worker's own value system.
- Involvement of the worker always changes the family's system.
- Anyone who plays a part in the problem system can be as much a part of the system as the family is.
- Changes in the professional system or decision making often reflect shifts in the family system.
- Workers always need to be aware of issues of race, culture, gender and other difference.
- Such differences become structured in terms of power and need to be located and understood, for example gender roles within families.
- Clarification and development of appropriate boundaries can promote change.
- There is value in introducing a different approach in long-term work in order to promote change. Workers as well as families can become stuck.
- Joint or co-work can be a helpful and economic method to promote change.
- The dynamics of the family may be acutely experienced in the co-work relationship.
- Assessment and working with families to promote change sometimes needs to be distinct activities, although there is commonly an element of each in the other.
- The dilemmas for a social worker carrying a dual role, for example child protection and family problem solving, need careful consideration. The roles may not always be compatible.
- The social worker's position of neutrality is a complex matter in relation to agency function.
- Monitoring personal responses to the work is an important component of reflective practice.

A management perspective

Part 3:
Implications for policy and practice

A management perspective

Patrick Kidner

When I was invited, as a former social work manager in a London local authority, to write this concluding chapter, the brief was quite straightforward. It was, in a nutshell, to explore the implications of the case studies for policy and practice from the perspective of a practice supervisor and middle manager. Not having supervised practice for some years, I consulted a former colleague who was until recently a first-line manager, and asked her to comment on the early drafts. Together we had extensive experience in local authority social work, the voluntary sector, probation service and social work teaching.

The task proved very challenging, especially bearing in mind that we had been given, so to speak, 'the last word' in writing the concluding chapter. Inevitably it has been necessary to be selective. From the wealth of case material in addition to the commentaries, we have chosen several issues which seemed important and worth pursuing. We were aware of the fact that the students involved had not written with a view to publication but rather for their own learning. How different would their approach have been if they had been writing for a wider audience, including potential critics from the realms of academia and management?

In writing as they have, they provide us with a truly inside view of social work practice with children and families in the later 1990s. A less honest or more 'sanitised' account would have deprived the reader of some valuable insights into the stressful nature of the job and the difficulties faced by practitioners in attempting to develop their skills.

Nevertheless, the 'warts and all' approach prompts another set of questions in the context of the wider debate about social work and its place in the national psyche. Is there any other profession which so openly displays its limitations, as well as its success stories, in everyday practice? Is it wise for social workers to do so when their credibility and status are already subject to repeated attack by politicians and the media? And how would the average user make sense of these accounts? It is tempting to think that some may have judged the efforts of the practitioners less harshly than they did themselves.

Our task in this chapter is not so much to judge as to identify some key messages for practitioners and managers. A useful starting point is to acknowledge that the struggle for high quality reflective practice is not widely understood or supported in the realms of senior management or the political arena, and the closure of the Goldsmiths course may be symptomatic of this. In the prevailing climate of hostility towards social work, the authors of the case studies can be likened to heroic footsoldiers going 'over the top' under the banner of good practice, with limited covering fire and rather spasmodic encouragement from their superior officers.

If this is a fair analogy, what lessons can we draw from the case studies and commentaries, and what do they tell us about the state of professional practice as we enter the new millennium? Our comments can be grouped under three main headings:

- theory, research and the issue of effectiveness;
- dilemmas in the practitioner's role;
- support for reflective practice.

Theory, research and the issue of effectiveness

As one might expect of students on an academic course, the authors of the case studies draw on a wide range of material to illuminate their practice. They have evidently seized the opportunity both to re-visit concepts and ideas derived from basic training, and to explore some with which they were not previously familiar. There is excitement in the quest for coherence and meaning in situations of great confusion and complexity: a need for 'conceptual maps' so that practice can be viewed, as it were, from a distance which offers a broader picture and a sense of direction.

Such perspectives are important, whether the focus is on the inner world of a child or on a family's relationship with its professional network. It is unusual, as the studies suggest, for practitioners, or indeed their supervisors, to feel equally comfortable in both arenas or to manage to keep them both simultaneously in mind, but it is an ideal which the commentators uphold and should be a recurring theme of skilled supervision.

Leaving aside our personal bias, what is our 'management perspective' on the use of the material by the case study authors? At the risk of stating the obvious, we should start by affirming the value of the reflection process itself. This is not just an intellectual exercise designed to satisfy course requirements but a chance to apply current theory and research to some common experiences in practice. From this perspective, it is the process itself which is more important to the busy manager than the choice of material, of which they may in any case have limited knowledge.

Nevertheless, the studies also illustrate a common bias among practitioners, in placing more emphasis on the process and method of intervention rather than its purpose and outcome: in other words, on the whole issue of effectiveness. This is a surprising feature of the studies, given the growing body of literature and relevant research, but it is not difficult to suggest why practitioners might be reluctant to address it. Perhaps they are indeed 'the herbalists of the helping professions' who "just know from personal experience which approaches work and which not, though not necessarily why and how" (Sheldon and McDonald, 1993, p 211).

To be fair, none of the authors displays this kind of complacency and several are prepared to acknowledge shortcomings in evaluating their work. The difficulty lies more in their struggle to define clear aims and hence potential outcomes in a way which lends itself to 'objective' appraisal. Stephen Kitchman is a notable exception. When the Dray family is referred to him, he is invited by an outgoing colleague "to assess the need for and ... input family support as appropriate". His commendable response to this rather global injunction is to draft a written agreement with the parents, listing tasks and responsibilities and including a commitment to review progress on a given date. Unfortunately he is then thwarted by the sudden and unexpected move of the family, so we are left to guess at the impact of his intervention.

Michael O'Dempsey presents a more finished piece of work with Amos and Christopher, and sets out an explicit list of goals which interestingly omits the possibility of reuniting the children with their mother. This is in fact achieved but is not presented as a consequence or outcome of the work, however desirable it may have been. In other examples, objectives are implicit in the text or in the context of the work; are framed in terms of assessing issues or relationships; or must be deduced from the author's evaluation.

An important aspect of day-to-day practice in a busy agency is illustrated in these examples, namely that it is rarely possible to view social work intervention as a discrete process with predetermined time-scales and objectives. More often than not, it is part of a series of interrelated activities effected by different parties, in which both factors need constant review as new information emerges and as priorities change for practitioner and team. Kate Wilson alludes to this in her reference to Mary Cody's post-adoption work and the apparent shift from 'empowerment' to 'achieving an understanding of Eve's feelings' as the stated purpose.

The notion of 'outcome' in social work practice is no less problematic as this definition from a study of looked after children suggests:

> ... outcomes cannot be regarded as free-standing states waiting to be discovered and evaluated; they are products of selection, shaped by the interplay of different interests, assumptions and aspirations. (DoH, 1995, p 41)

This complexity is reflected in Veronique Faure's evaluation of her work with Carol, Anna and Khadia and in the response of the commentators. The purpose is stated as an assessment of the risks to Khadia arising from increased contact with her father (who is also her mother's step-brother). Acknowledging that there are 'no final resolutions', Faure is self-critical and anxious about the impact of the work, which seemed to precipitate Anna's ejection from home by her mother. On the other hand, she recognises the potential value to Anna in being more independent, assertive and aware of her needs.

Sigurd Reimers takes issue with her about her sense of failure and endorses the need for greater emotional distance between Carol and Anna. Jane Dutton also applauds her for "working positively with uncertainty and ambiguity", while underlining the value of joint work and of careful preparation for such an intervention. The question which is not directly addressed by either the commentators or Faure herself, despite her stated purpose, is whether Khadia is at greater or less risk as a result of her mother's ejection from home. It is indeed difficult to maintain a sharp focus in such a shifting environment, especially when clinical perspectives such as Reimers may differ, in emphasis at least, from those of an agency with its reputation to protect.

So what do these examples tell us about the dilemmas for practitioners in defining objectives clearly and evaluating outcomes? For a start it may help, as Reimers sugests, to "look over our shoulders" in a systemic way and to recognise the range of vested interests competing for our attention: needs of the child as against those of the parent; professional values as against agency policy; clinical perspectives as against priorities of management – to name but a few.

What is far more difficult is to make some kind of choice by naming objectives explicitly and by defining priorities between them. Reimers seems almost to caution against this very process in family work, preferring the notion of 'explorer' to that of 'expert' as a basis for effecting therapeutic change. In the same vein, he urges Patrick Lonergan not to be "too wedded to a particular outcome" in reviewing his work with a very dependent family. Nevertheless, in his comment on Cody's family assessment, he also recognises the existence of 'inbuilt conflicts of interest' arising from the task entrusted by the state to the social worker. This is likely to limit the potential impact of social work intervention but to a lesser extent if the conflicts are openly acknowledged.

Here, then, is an initial reason for practitioners, especially those with clear statutory powers, to hesitate in defining objectives. For a start, it means accepting limitations in their therapeutic powers and options, as Faure, for example, concedes in her evaluation of the work with Sarah.

Second, it makes practitioners vulnerable to management 'interference' when objectives are not felt to comply with agency policy, or to criticism when they are not achieved. Cody's stated intention of completing her home study in six months rather than, say, three or four, could invite her agency to question whether such a lengthy process is either necessary or appropriate. Kitchman's written agreement and commitment to review ensures that both he and the family support officer can be held to account for the resources employed in the work, not only by the agency but by the family as well.

Third, explicit definitions of objectives can bring sharply into focus differences in the values and aspirations of the various parties, including service users, practitioners and their managers. It has been suggested for example that users tend to favour subjective and qualitative factors in considering outcomes, in contrast to the objective, and ideally measurable, factors preferred by service managers (Turner, 1998). The wish 'to have more control over one's life', for example, may be an aspiration with which as many practitioners as users will identify, but is difficult to translate into a performance target for their managers.

In such 'quicksands' of practice (for this is surely how it sometimes feels), there can be no panacea for the dilemmas of practitioners seeking to intervene with purpose and clarity. The risk of being swamped by overwhelming demands and unrealistic aspirations should be a good incentive for them to struggle with these issues. Current research also offers encouragement to practitioners and supervisors alike, not least in the resounding endorsement for 'sensitive and informed professional/client relationships' and 'effective supervision and training' as two of the preconditions for effective practice in child protection (DoH, 1995). (It was surprising that this seminal document was not mentioned in any of the case studies.)

Again, the pessimistic results of early studies into the effectiveness of practice have been overtaken by the findings of more recent investigations. One review of 87 studies carried out between 1979 and 1991 concluded that 75% demonstrated "clearly positive results testifying to the effectiveness of social work" (Sheldon and McDonald, 1993, p 215). The conclusion of a separate article concerning the same review was more specific in stating that "many studies with positive outcomes (whatever the specific approach employed) contain clear openly stated objectives – shared with clients – and an explicit expectation that results will accrue within a given time period" (Macdonald et al, 1992, p 636). Purposeful practice, well grounded in research and supported by skilled supervision, is surely the best antidote to predatory managers with an eye on budget savings, and a sceptical public seeking scapegoats for the ills of society.

Dilemmas in the practitioner's role

A second major theme of the case studies concerns the variety of roles and strategies employed by practitioners in attempting to work constructively with children and their families. Almost invariably there is a substantial network of other professionals with whom a coherent approach must be established, but differences emerge in the way this is done and in the practitioners' understanding of their own role and tasks. Choices are made in the allocation of tasks, in the priorities they are given and in the way they are carried out. For managers and supervisors, the challenge is to be aware of these choices, to participate in making them when appropriate, and to understand their implications for service users, for practitioners and for the agency itself.

If there is one overarching message from the case studies, it is a positive one about the benefits of diversity in choice of working methods. The sample is too small to form a basis for generalising about the comparative merits of particular methods, but some of the material calls for additional comment from a management perspective.

First, it is important to keep in perspective the familiar debate about the difficulties of combining key worker responsibilities or case management with direct work. Lonergan and Kitchman demonstrate the possibilities both in their work with whole families and with children, as O'Dempsey does with Amos and Christopher. From a supervisory point of view, extra time must be conceded for the work itself and for reflection and supervision or consultation; but the overall demand on resources is probably less than would arise if another worker had to be coopted. From the child or family's perspective, of course, this model also has the advantage of limiting the number of professionals with a stake in their affairs. The positive outcomes in some of these cases suggest that any conflict of roles is manageable, if at times uncomfortable.

By contrast, the 'split role' model, exemlified here by Faure and Michael Atkinson, is likely to be more demanding of resources in the short term but may have compensating advantages. In her family assessment, Faure works simultaneously in sessions with the allocated social worker and brings a new perspective to the situation, as both commentators note appreciatively. However, Dutton especially underlines the importance of careful preparation for this type of joint work, and might have added some reference to the role of supervision in that process. In practice, supervision of joint work can be time-consuming (specific to one case) and difficult to organise, especially if the practitioners are from different teams or agencies.

Against this, Reimers and Dutton emphasise that some families can benefit from the introduction of a second practitioner if the joint work is properly planned and differences, for example of race, power and gender, can be usefully shared as part of the therapeutic process. For practitioners too, there will often be times when immediate access to a co-worker, or perhaps to a live supervisor behind a one-way screen, can be invaluable to confidence and morale. But social services managers are often faced with stark choices about how personnel will be deployed, which is one reason why the opportunities for working jointly in that setting are relatively few.

Working jointly does not always mean simultaneously, as Faure demonstrates in her separate sessions with four-year-old Sarah. In this third model, the practitioner has no case management responsibility and is free to focus on the individual needs of the child, with the support of specialist consultation. Taking Wilson's point about the importance of 'integration', it would have been helpful to know how Faure's work related to that of the allocated social worker, and what preparations they made to coordinate their activity. In Atkinson's case, he convened a meeting with the allocated social worker and other professionals before embarking on sessions with the family.

From a management perspective, two key themes emerge from this analysis. First, there must be continuing attention to the development of direct work skills, as Wilson and Helen Martyn suggest, from qualifying courses onwards, if services to children and families are to become genuinely child-centred. Case managers without such skills are likely to jeopardise the child's right to participate in decisions affecting their lives. Second, the impact of any direct work is likely to be much less, or even adverse, if it is not fully integrated with the work of other services. In other words, good case management is, or should be, a precondition for effective direct work, even if it is sometimes uncomfortable trying to combine these roles.

For local authority fieldworkers, the burden is particularly acute, bearing in mind the effects of adverse publicity about notorious cases, and the growing expectations that they will meet exacting standards of care at a time of continuing change and often declining resources. The recent invitation to BASW and to the Local Government Association to undertake a study of the fieldworker's role, is welcome and timely (Utting, 1998). One hopes that their brief will extend to the adequacy of basic training and staff development opportunities in the relevant agencies.

Support for reflective practice

If the role of practitioners is complex and evolving, so too is that of their supervisors, and in this final section we consider what lessons the case studies offer for the development of practice supervision in the next few years.

It is difficult to know, as it was not part of the brief, precisely what part supervision played in each of the studies. Reference to the stressful and complex nature of the work (and none of the cases were particularly exceptional in this respect) are indicative of the practitioners' need, but evidence about the contribution of supervision is at best patchy. In some cases it is hardly mentioned and in others it is seen as crucial, often complemented by off-line consultation with a variety of specialists.

In her work with Sarah, for example, Faure valued the supervision from her course coordinator and consultation from a child psychologist. Together they provided 'a safe space' to evaluate her practice and to manage the feelings, both conscious and unconscious, which the sessions aroused. This is also the focus of O'Dempsey's 'supervision' by a child pychologist and Cody's by her agency supervisor, although she too would like further specialist consultation.

What these examples highlight – and something that is only too obvious in many social services departments today – is that supervisors rarely have the time, skills or experience to support the kind of practice exemplified here. Just as practitioners need to strike a balance between case management and direct work, so also must supervisors attend to the whole workload ('the inquisitorial function') as well as to particular cases which are causing anxiety ('the empathic-containing function') (Rushton and Nathan, 1996). The evidence from several of the studies is that practitioners will often need to look beyond their regular supervisor for support with the second function, and are more likely to find it outside their own management line, if not in a different agency altogether.

It is not necessary to look far for the reasons behind this trend. Increasing specialisation in recent years and targeting of high priority groups for services has ensured that most practitioners carry an undiluted workload of complex and demanding cases. Changes in policy and legislation in the wake of child abuse enquiries have led to repeated reorganisation, and in particular to increased reliance on market forces as a means of coordinating services (Barker, 1996).

Separation of purchaser and provider roles, and devolution of budgets to team manager level, have placed new demands on middle managers, including heightened responsibility for resource allocation. To their other skills, they have had to add the ability to handle increasing quantities of management and financial information. A new managerial culture has emerged in response to these developments, valuing competition between managers and teams in achieving specified targets, and offering the rewards (and sanctions) of performance related pay.

For many team managers and practice supervisors, it has been difficult to reconcile the values implicit in these changes with their existing commitments to the notion of 'needs led' services. If they over-identify with practitioners, they risk becoming collusive in their rejection of the agency's values; conversely, they may become persecutory in the eyes of practitioners if they adopt the new culture with too much enthusiasm – 'suckers or bastards' as earlier commentators have described them (Mattinson and Sinclair, 1979).

The case studies suggest that the second option may be in the ascendant, to the detriment of supervision and the needs of practitioners. Further evidence of this tendency can be found in a qualitative survey of Inner London team managers who linked their own limitations as supervisors to the absence of consistent support from their line managers. They also felt training away from the work setting was necessary to assimilate knowledge about new developments and research in child protection (Rushton and Nathan, 1996).

Similar sentiments were expressed by practitioners who had completed the advanced courses at Goldsmiths and the Maudsley Hospital. They were unanimous in preferring a college-based course, shared with colleagues from other agencies, and over a third expressed dissatisfaction with the opportunities to apply what they had learned on return to their agency (Rushton and Martyn, 1993). Another study of three social services departments by NISW found that teams were preoccupied with top-down information, and that there was an absence of structures and policies to support practice (Kearney and Rosen, 1999).

This rather pessimistic picture is all the more surprising when set against the recommendations of numerous child abuse inquiries and SSI inspections in recent years. There is a real danger that the creative role of practitioners will be stifled by increasingly bureacratic and prescriptive forms of management, if more attention is not urgently given to the support and development of first-line managers and practice supervisors.

How can these pervasive and damaging trends be reversed, and are there more hopeful signs for reflective practice on the horizon? It is tempting to believe that centrally driven initiatives, like the 'Looked After Children' system and Quality Protects, will provide an impetus for improving practice by adopting a more systematic approach to information gathering, and by setting targets and performance indicators which will become a benchmark for all local authorities. The demise of CCETSW and creation of the new General Social Care Council may also afford opportunities to set new standards for practitioners and supervisors at a national level, especially if a higher proportion of training funds can be secured for post-qualifying courses.

But the message of the case studies and of the discussion they have prompted here is that social services departments are still ambivalent about the skills required of practitioners. Until directors and senior managers show greater interest in the development of practice in their own departments, and create expectations about learning on or off the job, it will be difficult to recruit and retain the highly skilled practitioners they require.

Acknowledgement

I am indebted to Liz Green, formerly team manager in Wandsworth Social Services Department and currently area manager for the NSPCC, for her advice on this chapter and comments on the early drafts.

References and further reading

Adcock, M., Dubois, D. and Small, A. (1988) 'Ending relationships successfully', in J.Aldgate and J. Simmonds (eds) *Direct work with children. A guide for social work practitioners*, London: Batsford/BAAF.

Ahmed, S., Cheetham, J. and Small, J. (eds) (1986) *Social work with black children and their families*, London: Batsford/BAAF.

Aldgate, J. and Simmonds, J. (eds) (1988) *Direct work with children. A guide for social work practitioners*, London: Batsford/BAAF.

Aldridge, J. and Becker, S. (1993) *Children who care*, Loughborough: Department of Social Sciences, Loughborough University.

Anderson, H. and Goolishian, H. (1988) 'Human systems as linguistic systems', *Family Process*, vol 27, pp 371-93.

Asen, E. (1995) *Family therapy for everyone*, London: BBC Books.

Asen, E. (1996) Lecture notes, Postgraduate Diploma in Advanced Social Work, Goldsmiths College, University of London.

Asen, E. and Tomson, P. (1992) *Family solutions in family practice*, Lancaster: Quay Publishing.

Axline, V. (1947) *Play therapy*, New York, NY: Ballantine.

Axline, V. (1964) *Dibs: In search of self*, London: Gollancz.

Balloch, S. (ed) (1998) *Outcomes of social care,* London: NISW.

Barnes, G. Gorell (1985) 'Systems theory and family theory', in M. Rutter and L. Hersov (eds) *Child and adolescent psychiatry*, 2nd edn, Oxford: Blackwell.

Barnes, G. Gorell (1995) 'The intersubjective mind', in M. Yelloly and M. Henkel (eds) *Learning and teaching in social work: Towards reflective practice*, London: Jessica Kingsley.

Barker, R.W. (1996) 'Child protection, public services and the chimera of market force efficiency', *Children and Society*, vol 10, no 1, pp 28-39.

Bateson, G. (1972) *Steps to an ecology of mind*, London: Paladin.

Batty, D. (ed) (1989) *Working with children*, London: BAAF.

Biehal, N., Clayden, J., Stein, M. and Wade, R. (1995) *Moving on: Young people and leaving care schemes*, London: HMSO.

Blom-Cooper, L. (1985) *A child in trust*, London: London Borough of Brent.

Blom-Cooper, L., Harding, J. and Milton, E. (1987) *A child in mind: Protection of children in a responsible society*, London: Greenwich Social Services Department.

Bohannen, P. (1971) *Divorce and after*, New York, NY: Doubleday.

Bowlby, J. (1969) *Attachment and loss*, vol 1, New York, NY: Basic Books.

Bowlby, J. (1971) *Attachment*, Harmondsworth: Penguin.

Bowlby, J. (1979) *The making and breaking of affectional bonds*, London: Tavistock.

Bowlby, J. (1980) *Attachment and loss*, vol 3, London: Hogarth Press.

Bowlby, J. (1988) *A secure base*, London: Tavistock/Routledge.

Brand, D. (1999) *Accountable care: Developing the General Social Care Council*, York: Jospeh Rowntree Foundation.

Bretherton, I. (1991) 'The roots and growing points of attachment theory', in C.M. Parkes, J. Stevenson Hinde and P. Marris (eds) *Attachment across the life cycle,* London: Routledge.

Bridge Child Care Consultancy Service (1995) *Paul: Death through neglect*, London: Bridge Child Care Consultancy Service.

Briere, J.N. (1992) *Child abuse trauma: Theory and treatment of the lasting effect,* Newbury Park, California, CA: Sage Publications.

Briere, J. and Runtz, M. (1993) 'Childhood sexual abuse: long term sequelae and implications for psychological assessment', *Journal of Interpersonal Violence*, vol 8, no 3, pp 312-30.

Briggs, S. (1992) 'Child observation and social work training', *Journal of Social Work Practice,* vol 6, no 1, pp 49-61.

Brodzinsky, D. and Schechter, M. (eds) (1990) *The psychology of adoption*, New York, NY: Oxford University Press.

Brown, A. and Bourne, I. (1996) *The social work supervisor*, Buckingham: Open University Press.

Buchsbaum, H., Toth, S., Clyman, R., Cicchetti, D. and Emde, R. (1992) 'The use of narrative story stem technique with maltreated children', *Development & Psychotherapy*, vol 4, pp 603-25.

Burck, C. and Speed, B. (1995) *Gender, power and relationships,* London: Routledge.

Burnham, J. (1986) *Family therapy: First steps towards a systemic approach*, London: Routledge.

Burnham, J. and Harris, Q. (1997) 'Emerging ethnicity: a tale of three cultures', in K. Dwivedi and V. Varma (eds) *Meeting the needs of ethnic minority children*, London: Jessica Kingsley.

Byng-Hall, J. (1995) 'Creating a family science base: some implications of attachment theory for family therapy', *Family Process,* vol 34, no 1, pp 45-58.

Byng-Hall, J. and Hinde, J. Stevenson (1991) 'Attachment relationships within a family system', *Infant Mental Health Journal,* vol 12, no 3, pp 187-200.

Carpenter, J. (1996) 'Family therapy and empowerment', in P. Parsloe (ed) *Pathways to empowerment*, Birmingham: Venture Press.

Carrol, J. (1994) 'The protection of children exposed to marital violence', *Child Abuse Review*, vol 3, no 1, pp 6-14.

Carrol, J. (1998) *Introduction to therapeutic play*, Oxford: Blackwell Science.

Carter, E. and McGoldrick, M. (1980) *The family life cycle*, London: Gardener.

Cattenach, A. (1992) *Play therapy with abused children*, London: Jessica Kingsley.

Cattenach, A. (1994) *Play therapy: Where the sky meets the underworld*, London: Jessica Kingsley.

CCETSW (Central Council for Education and Training in Social Work) (1992) *Education and training in the personal social services. A framework for continual professional development*, Paper 31 (revised), London: CCETSW.

CCETSW (1995) *Assuring quality in the Diploma in Social Work – 1. Rules and requirements for the DipSW*, Paper 30, revised 2nd edn, London: CCETSW.

Cheetham, J., Fuller, R., McIvor, G. and Petch, A. (1992) *Evaluating social work effectiveness*, Buckingham: Open University Press.

Cleaver, H., Unell, I. and Aldgate, J. (1999) *Children's needs: Parenting capacity*, London: The Stationery Office.

Corden, J. and Shoot, M. Preston (1987) *Contracts in social work*, Aldershot: Gower.

Corrigan, P. and Leonard, P. (1978) *Social work practice under capitalism: A marxist approach,* London: Macmillan.

Dale, P. (1988) *Dangerous families*, London: Tavistock.

Dallos, R.(1991) *Family belief systems, therapy and change,* Buckingham: Open University Press.

Dimmock, B. and Dungworth, D. (1983) 'Creating manoeuverability for family systems therapists in social services departments', *Journal of Family Therapy*, vol 5, pp 53-69.

Dockar-Drysdale, B. (1968) 'The process of symbolisation observed among emotionally deprived children in theraputic schools', in R.J.N. Todd (ed) *Disturbed children*, London: Longman.

Dockar-Drysdale, B. (1990) *The provision of primary experience: Winnicottian work with children and adolescents*, London: Free Association Books.

Department of Health (DoH) (1988) *Protecting children. A guide for social workers undertaking a comprehensive assessment*, London: HMSO.

DoH (1991a) *Child abuse. A study of inquiry reports 1980-1989*, London: HMSO.

DoH (1991b) *Patterns and outcomes in child placement. Messages from current research and their implications*, London: HMSO.

DoH (1992) *A study of local authority decision making about public law applications*, Court orders study December 1992, London: Department of Health Social Services Inspectorate.

DoH (1993) *Children Act report 1992*, London: HMSO.

DoH (1994) *Children Act report 1993*, London: HMSO.

DoH (1995) *Child protection: Messages from research*, London: HMSO.

DoH (1996) *Protecting children: A guide for social workers undertaking a comprehensive assessment*, London: HMSO.

DoH (1998a) *Modernising social services*, London: The Stationery Office.

DoH (1998b) *Quality Protects: Framework for action plans*, London: DoH.

DoH (2000) *Framework for the assessment of children in need and their families*, London: The Stationery Office.

Dominelli, L. (1988) *Anti-racist social work*, London: BASW/Macmillan.

Donley, G. (1993) 'Attachment and the emotional unit', *Family Process*, vol 32, no 1, pp 3-20.

Downes, C. (1992) *Separation revisited*, Aldershot: Ashgate.

Driver, E. and Droisen, A. (1989) *Child sexual abuse: Feminist perspectives*, London: Macmillan.

Dungworth, D. and Reimers, S. (1984) 'Using family therapy in social services departments', in A. Treacher and J. Carpenter (eds) *Using family therapy: A guide for practitioners in different professional settings*, Oxford: Blackwell.

Fahlberg, V. (1981a) *Attachment and separation*, London: BAAF.

Fahlberg, V. (1981b) *Helping children when they must move*, London: BAAF.

Fahlberg, V. (1988) *Fitting the pieces together*, London: BAAF.

Fahlberg, V. (1994) *A child's journey through placement*, London: BAAF.

Finkelhor, D. (1984) *Child sexual abuse: new theory and research*, New York, NY: Free Press.

Galley, J. (1988) 'Permanancy planning for older children in care', in J. Aldgate and J. Simmonds (eds) *Direct work with children*, London: Batsford/BAAF.

Gelles, R. and Cornell, C. (1990) *Intimate violence in families*, London: Sage Publications.

Gil, E. (1991) *The healing power of play*, New York, NY: Guildford Press.

Glaser, D. (1995) 'Emotional abuse experiences', in P. Reder and C. Lucey (eds) *Assessment of parenting: Psychiatric and psychological contributions*, London: Routledge.

Glaser, D. (1996) Course notes, unpublished, Postgraduate Diploma in Advanced Social Work, Goldsmiths College, University of London.

Glaser, D. and Frosh, S. (1991) *Child sexual abuse*, London: Macmillan.

Glaser, D., Prior, V. and Lynch, M. (1994) *Messages from children: Children's evaluations of the professional response to child sexual abuse*, London: NCH Action for Children.

Goffman, E. (1968) *Stigma: Notes on the management of spoiled identity*, Harmondsworth: Penguin.

Goldner, V., Penn, P., Sheinberg, M. and Walker, G. (1990) 'Love and violence: gender paradoxes in volatile attachments', *Family Process*, vol 29, pp 343-64.

Goodrich, T.J. et al (1988) *Feminist family therapy: A casebook*, New York, NY: Norton.

Goodrich, W., Fullerton, C., Yates, B. and Berman, L. (1990) 'The residential treatment of severly disturbed adolescent adoptees', in D.M. Brodzinsky and M.D. Schechter (eds) *The psychology of adoption*, New York, NY: Oxford University Press.

Guerney, L. (1984) 'Client centred (non directive) play therapy', in C. Schaefer and K. O'Connor (eds) *Handbook of play therapy*, New York, NY: Wiley.

Haley, J. (1976) *Problem solving therapy*, New York, NY: Harper Colophon.

Haley, J. (1980) *Leaving home*, New York, NY: McGraw Hill.

Harding, T. and Beresford, P. (1996) *The standards we expect: What service users and carers want from social services workers*, London: NISW.

Hartman, A. (1979) *Finding families: An ecological approach to family assessment in adoption*, London: Sage Publications.

Hawkins, P. and Shohet, R. (1989) *Supervision in the helping professions*, Buckingham: Open University Press.

Hinde, J. Stevenson (1990) 'Attachment within family systems: an overview', *Infant Mental Health Journal* vol 11, no 3, pp 218-27.

Hjelle, L.A. and Ziegler, D.J. (1985) *Personality theories: Basic assumptions, research and implications*, New York, NY: McGraw Hill.

Hoffman, L. (1990) 'Constructing realities: an art of lenses', *Family Process*, vol 29, pp 1-12.

Holman, A. (1983) *Family assessment tools for understanding and intervention*, Beverly Hills, California, CA: Sage Publications.

Holmes, J. (1993) *John Bowlby and attachment theory*, London: Routledge.

Howe, D. (1987) *An introduction to social work theory*, Aldershot: Aldgate.

Howe, D. (1995) *Attachment theory for social work practice*, London: Macmillan.

Hughes, S., Berger, M. and Wright, L. (1978) 'The family life cycle and clinical intervention', *Journal of Marriage and Family Counselling*, vol 5, pp 33-40.

Iwaniec, D. (1995) *The emotionally abused and neglected child*, Chichester: Wiley.

Jacobs, M. (1988) *Psychodynamic counselling in action*, London: Sage Publications.

Jewett, C. (1984) *Helping children cope with separation and loss*, London: Batsford/BAAF.

Jones, E. (1991) *Working with adult survivors of child sexual abuse*, London: Karnac Books.

Jordan, B. (1979) *Helping in social work,* London: Routledge.

Katz, L., Spoonemore, N. and Robinson, C. (1994) *Concurrent planning from permanancy planning to permanancy action*, Lutheran Social Services, Washington and Idaho.

Kearney, P. (ed) (1999) *The management of practice expertise. Project report*, London: NISW.

Kearney, P. and Rosen, G. (1998) 'Shaping routine', *Community Care,* 26 November, pp 32-3.

Kirk, D. (1984) *Shared fate: A theory and method of adoptive relations*, Washington, DC: Ben-Simon Publications.

Kitchman, S. (1996) 'The child speaks: views of children about child protection social work', Research project, unpublished, Postgraduate Diploma in Advanced Social Work, Goldsmiths College, University of London, July.

Kramer, S. (1995) 'What are fathers for?', in C. Burck and B. Speed (eds) *Gender, power and relationships,* London: Routledge.

Laing, R.D. (1969) *Intervention in social situations*, London: Association of Family Caseworkers/Philadelphia Association Ltd.

Landreth, G. (1991) *Play therapy: The art of the relationship,* Muncie, IA: Accelerated Development Inc.

Laplanche, J. and Pontalis, J.B. (1992) 'The language of psychoanalysis', Course notes, 'Child sexual abuse within the family: an inter-agency approach', Portman and Tavistock Clinic.

Le Riche, P. and Tanner, K. (eds) (1998) *Observation and its application to social work: Rather like breathing*, London: Jessica Kingsley.

Macdonald, G., Sheldon, B. and Gillespie, J. (1992) 'Contemporary studies of the effectiveness of social work', *British Journal of Social Work,* vol 22, no 6, pp 615-43.

MacLeod, M. and Saraga, P. (1987) 'Abuse of trust', *Journal of Social Work Practice,* vol 3, no 1, pp 71-9.

McMahan, L. (1992) *The handbook of play therapy*, London: Tavistock/ Routledge.

Main, M. (1991) 'Metacognitive knowledge, metacognitive monitoring and singular (coherent) versus multiple (incoherent) models of attachment', in C.M. Parkes, J. Stevenson Hinde and P. Parkes, *Attachment across the life cycle,* London: Routledge.

Manor, O. (1984) *Family work in action,* London: Tavistock.

Marris, P. (1974) *Loss and change*, New York, NY: Random House.

Mattinson, J. (1992) *The reflection process in casework supervision*, London: Tavistock.

Mattinson, J. and Sinclair, I. (1979) *Mate and stalemate*, Oxford: Blackwell.

Menzies, I. (1970) *The functioning of social systems as a defence against anxiety*, London: Tavistock Institute.

Miller, A. (1993) *The drama of being a child*, London: Virago Press.

Miller, A.C. and Perelberg, R.J. (1990) *Gender and power in families*, London: Routledge.

Minuchin, S. (1974) *Families and family therapy*, London: Tavistock.

Minuchin, S. and Fishman, H.C. (1981) *Techniques of family therapy*, Cambridge, MA: Harvard University Press.

Morgan, S. and Righton, P. (1989) *Child care: Concerns and conflict*, London: Hodder and Stoughton.

Morris, J. (2000) *Having someone who cares: Barriers to change in the public care of children*, York/London: Joseph Rowntree Foundation/National Childrens Bureau.

Muncie, J. and Sapsford, R. (1993) 'Issues in the study of the family', in J. Muncie, M. Wetherell, M. Langan, R. Dallos and A. Cochran (eds) *Understanding the family,* London: Sage Publications.

NCH Action for Children (1994) *The hidden victims: Children and domestic violence,* London: NCH Action for Children.

NSPCC (1997) *Turning points: A resource for communicating with children,* Leicester: NSPCC.

NSPCC, Barnardo's and University of Bristol (1998) *Making an impact: Children and domestic violence,* Leicester: NSPCC.

NSPCC, NDCS and Way Ahead Consultancy (1994) *ABCD: Abuse and children who are disabled,* Leicester: NSPCC.

NSPCC, University of Sheffield (2000) *The child's world: Assessing children's needs,* Leicester: NSPCC.

O'Hagan, K. and Dillenburger, K. (1995) *The abuse of women within child care work,* Buckingham: Open University Press.

Open University (1990) *Working with children and young people,* Buckingham: Open University Press.

Pagelow, M. (1981) *Woman battering. Victims and their experiences,* Beverly Hills, California, CA: Sage Publications.

Palazzoli, M., Cecchin, G., Prata, C. and Boscolo, L. (1978) *Paradox and counter-paradox,* New York, NY: Aronson.

Palazzoli, M., Cecchin, G., Prata, C. and Boscolo, L. (1980) 'Hypothesising, circularity, neutrality: three guidelines for the conductor of the session', *Family Process,* vol 19, pp 3-12.

Parkes, C.M. (1988) *Bereavement: Studies of grief in adult life,* Harmondsworth: Penguin.

Parkes, C.M., Hinde, J. Stevenson and Marris, P. (1991) *Attachment across the life cycle,* London: Routledge.

Parker, R., Ward, H., Jackson, S., Aldgate, J. and Wedge, P. (eds) (1991) *Looking after children: Assessing outcomes in child care,* London: HMSO.

Parton, N. (ed) (1997) *Child protection and family support,* London: Routledge.

Preston Shoot, M. (1994) *Practising social work,* London: Macmillan.

Pringle, M.K. (1975) *The needs of children*, London: Hutchinson.

Reder, P. and Duncan, S. (1995) 'Closure, covert warnings and escalating child abuse', *Child Abuse and Neglect*, vol 19, no 12, pp 1517-21.

Reder, P. and Lucey, C. (1995) *Assessment of parenting: Psychiatric and psychological contributions,* London: Routledge.

Reder, P., Duncan, S. and Gray, M. (1993) *Beyond blame: Child abuse tragedies revisited,* London: Routledge.

Redgrave, K. (1987) *Child's play. Direct work with the deprived child,* Cheadle: Boys and Girls Welfare Society.

Rees, S. and Wallace, A. (1982) *Verdicts on social work*, London: Edward Arnold.

Reimers, S. and Street, E. (1993) 'Using family therapy in child and adolescent services', in J. Carpenter and A. Treacher (eds) *Using family therapy in the 1990s: A guide for practitioners in different professional settings*, Oxford: Blackwell.

Reimers, S. and Treacher, A. (1995) *Introducing user-friendly family therapy*, London: Routledge.

Rogers, W., Hevey, D., Roche, J. and Ashe, E. (1992) *Child abuse and neglect: Facing the challenge*, 2nd edn, Buckingham: Open University Press.

Rosen, G. (ed) (2000) *Integrity: The organisation and the first line manager,* London: NISW.

Rosenbaum, A. and O'Leary, K.D. (1981) 'Marital violence: characteristics of abusive couples', *Journal of Consulting and Clinical Psychology,* vol 49, pp 63-71.

Rushton, A. and Martyn, H. (1993) *Learning for advanced practice,* Paper 31.1, London: CCETSW.

Rushton, A. and Nathan, J. (1996) 'The supervision of child protection work', *British Journal of Social Work*, vol 26, no 3, pp 357-74.

Rutter, M. (1972) *Maternal deprivation reassessed,* Harmondsworth: Penguin.

Rutter. M. (1999) 'Resilance concepts and findings: implications for family therapy', *Journal of Family Therapy*, vol 21, pp 119-44.

Rutter, M. and Hersov, L. (eds) (1985) *Child and adolescent psychiatry: Modern approaches*, 2nd edn, Oxford: Blackwell Scientific.

Ryan, T. and Walker, R. (1985) *Making life story books*, London: BAAF.

Ryan, V. and Wilson, K. (1996) *Case studies in non-directive play therapy*, London: Bailliere Tindall (reprinted 2000, London: Jessica Kingsley).

Ryan, V. and Wilson, K. (2000a) 'Conducting child assessments for court proceedings: the use of non-directive play therapy', *Clinical Child Psychology and Psychiatry*, vol 5, no 2, pp 267-79, April.

Ryan, V. and Wilson, K. (2000b) Using non-directive play therapy in court assessments: our response to Turner's legal commentary', *Clinical Child Psychology and Psychiatry*, vol 5, no 2, pp 282-3, April.

Sainsbury, E. (ed) (1994) *Working with children in need: Studies in complexity and challenge*, London: Jessica Kingsley.

Sainsbury, E., Nixon, S. and Phillips, D. (1982) *Social work in focus: Clients' and social workers' perceptions of long term work*, London: Routledge and Kegan Paul.

Salzberger, K. and Wittenberg, J. (1970) *Psychoanalytic insight and relationships: A Kleinian approach*, London: Routledge and Kegan Paul.

Sanford, L. (1991) *Strong at the broken places*, London: Virago Press.

Satir, V. (1972) *People making*, London: Souvenir Press.

Schon, D. (1987) *Educating the reflective practitioner*, San Francisco, CA: Jossey-Bass.

Schuff, G.H. and Asen, K.E. (1996) 'The disturbed parent and the disturbed family', in M. Coqfet, J. Webster and M. Seemen (eds) *Parental psychiatric disorder*, Cambridge: Cambridge University Press.

Segal, J. (1985) *Phantasy in everyday life: A psychoanalytic approach to understanding ourselves*, Harmondsworth: Penguin.

Sgroi, S. (1982) *A handbook of clinical intervention in child sexual abuse*, Lexington, MA: Lexington Books.

Shaver, K. (1985) *The attribution of blame*, London: Souvenir Press.

Sheldon, B. (1986) 'Social work effectiveness experiments: review and implications', *British Journal of Social Work*, vol 16, pp 223-42.

Sheldon, B. and MacDonald, G. (1993) 'Implications for practice of recent social work effectiveness research', *Practice*, vol 6 no 3.

Smale, G. (1999) *Managing change through innovation*, London: The Stationery Office.

Smale, G., Tuson, G. and Statham, D. (2000) *Social work and social problems: Working towards social inclusion and social change*, London: Macmillan.

Small, J. (1989) 'Transracial placements: conflicts and contradictions', in S. Morgan and P. Righton (eds) *Child care: Concerns and conflicts*, London: Hodder and Stoughton.

Smith, D. and Kingston, P. (1980) 'Live supervision without a one-way screen', *Journal of Family Therapy*, vol 2, pp 379-87.

Stein, M. (1997) *What works in leaving care*, Ilford: Barnardo's.

Stein, M. and Carey, K. (1986) *Leaving care*, Oxford: Blackwell.

Stewart, A., Friedman, S. and Koch, J. (1985) *Child development: A topical approach*, Chichester: Wiley.

Thoburn, J. (1990) *Success and failure in permanent family placement*, Aldershot: Gower/Averbury.

Tizard, B. (1987) *The care of young children. Implications of recent research*, London: Thomas Coram Foundation.

Treacher, A. (1995) 'Guidelines for user-friendly practice', in S. Reimers and A. Treacher, *Introducing user-friendly family therapy*, London: Routledge.

Treacher, A. and Carpenter, J. (1993) 'User-friendly family therapy', in J. Carpenter and A. Treacher (eds) *Using family therapy in the 1990s*, Oxford: Blackwell.

Triseliotis, J. (1983) 'Identity and security in long term fostering and adoption', *Adoption and Fostering*, vol 7, no 1, pp 22-31.

Trowell, J. and King, M. (1992) *Children's welfare and the law: The limits of legal intervention*, London: Sage Publications.

Trowell, J. and Miles, G. (1991) 'The contribution of observation training to professional development in social work', *Journal of Social Work Practice*, vol 5, no 1, pp 51-60.

Turner, M. (1998) 'The subjectivity of outcomes', in S. Balloch (ed) *Outcomes of social care*, London: NISW.

Utting, W. (1998) *People like us: Report of the review of the safeguards for children living away from home*, London: The Stationery Office.

VACSG (Violence Against Children Study Group) (1990) *Taking child abuse seriously*, London: Unwin Hyman.

Van der Kelk, B. (1987) *Psychological trauma*, Washington, DC: American Psychiatric Press.

Van der Kelk, B.A. and Kaddish, W. (1987) 'Amnesia, dissociation and the return of the repressed', in B. Van der Kelk *Psychological trauma*, Washington, DC: American Psychiatric Press.

Van Fleet, R. (1994) 'Filial therapy for adoptive children and parents', in K. O'Connor and C. Schaefer (eds) *Handbook of play therapy. Volume 2. Advances and innovations,* Chichester: Wiley.

Wallerstein, J. and Blakeslee, R. (1989) *Second chances: Men, women and children a decade after divorce*, London: Bantam Press.

Wallerstein, J. and Kelly, J. (1980) *Surviving the breakup: How children and parents cope with divorce*, New York, NY: Basic Books.

Wedge, P. and Thoburn, J. (1986) (eds) *Finding families for 'hard to place' children: Evidence from research*, London: BAAF.

West, J. (1996) *Child centred play therapy*, London: Arnold.

White, M. and Epston, D. (1990) *Narrative means to therapeutic ends,* New York, NY: Norton.

White, R., Carr, P. and Lowe, W. (1990) *A guide to the Children Act 1989,* Kent: Butterworth.

Williams, Lord (chair) (1996) *Childhood matters: report of the National Commission of Inquiry into the Prevention of Child Abuse*, London: The Stationery Office.

Wilson, K. (1992) 'The place of child observation in social work training', *Journal of Social Work Practice*, vol 6, no 1, pp 37–47.

Wilson, K., Kendrick, P. and Ryan, V. (1992) *Play therapy: A non-directive approach for children and adolescents,* London: Bailliere Tindall.

Winnicott, D. (1964) *The child, the family and the outside world,* Harmondsworth: Penguin.

Winnicott, D. (1984) 'Face to face with children', in *In touch with children*, London: BAAF.

Wyatt, G. and Powell, G. ((eds) 1988) *Lasting effects of child sexual abuse*, London: Sage Publications.

Wyre, R. (1987) *Working with sex abuse: Understanding sex offending*, Oxford: Perry.

Young, J. (1990) *Cognitive therapy for personality disorders: A schema focused approach*, Florida, FA: Professional Resource Exchange.

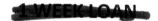